DEATH IS NOTHING TO FEAR

Better Living through the Philosophy of Epicurus

By the author of

Epicurus and the Pleasant Life

DEATH

IS NOTHING TO

FEAR

Better Living through the Philosophy of Epicurus

Haris Dimitriadis

Author-Publisher © Haris Dimitriadis, 2019

Text editors: Ben Way and Christie Moreton

Cover designer: Latte Goldstein

ISBN 978-1687729200

Visit the site
www.epicurusphilosophy.com

Dedicated to Epicurus in memory and admiration

Athens, July 2019

"So death, the most terrifying of ills, is nothing to us, since so long as we exist, death is not with us; but when death comes, then we do not exist. It does not then concern either the living or the dead, since for the former it is not, and the latter are no more."

—Epicurus, *Letter to Menoeceus*

ABOUT THE AUTHOR

Born in Greece, Haris studied Mathematics at the Aristotelian University of Thessaloniki, as well as Economics at the London School of Economics. His career spanned the business and banking industries, and he has now settled into retirement. Through climbing the corporate ladder, he found it brought little peace of mind and so he turned his attention to the philosophy of Epicurus. He has devoted the last two decades of his life to studying, reviving, and practicing the ancient Epicurean philosophy. Stunned by its effectiveness, he felt compelled to stimulate people's interest in and practice of the comprehensive and evidence-based philosophy of Epicurus in order to ameliorate their pain and live a pleasant life with health and peace of mind. In this context, he shared his learnings with the world by publishing *Epicurus and the Pleasant Life* in June 2017. The publication of *Death is Nothing to Fear* addresses the terror of the end of life in depth and offers effective means to cope with it, in view of the fact that this particular fear stops people from enjoying a pleasant life. Death is indeed the essential reminder of life. Only when we face up to it squarely can we take our time on this Earth seriously and make the most of it.

Currently, Haris—free from worries and fears—lives a pleasant life with his family and friends in Athens, enjoying reading, writing, philosophizing, sports, dancing, arts, and playing with his cherished granddaughter.

PREFACE

Dear reader,

Now is the time to reject cultural bias and heed the knowledge that Epicurus (341–270 BC) bestowed on us. Facing our own mortality and getting a firm grip on our fear of it are not only simple and straightforward achievements of the mind, but also indispensable to enjoying our lives. This clear-cut yet powerful assertion of Epicurus based on convincing arguments is contrary to the prevailing tradition supporting that we can live an eternal life under God's protection, through wealth, creativity, children, and societal customs.

Along this journey, we will explore rationales and evidence throughout the historical evolution of philosophy up to the time of Epicurus, the ancient Greek philosopher who laid the foundations for a philosophy of Nature. More specifically, it is the only philosophy that embraces the mortality of man and introduces pleasure as the inherent human guide to a happy life.

Contemporary society is characterized by a denial and fear of death. This behavior is usually subconscious and always difficult to overcome. In many ways, we are all influenced and even consciously trained to resist death. This is done by parents, medical professionals, politicians, teachers, religious leaders, and the media. Furthermore, the enemy is also often found within. Most of us retain self-destructive childhood experiences that lead us to deny our mortality. Indeed, as children we observe people falling ill or passing away and eventually come to realize that our parents and ourselves are also unable to sustain our lives forever. This understanding carries with it the fear of death that, being unable to cope with as children, we suppress in our memory. From that point the suppressed fear of death will unconsciously exert a continuous influence on our lives and remerge later as a terror whenever our life is in danger.

A straight resolute gaze at fatality is the communique of this monograph. We should meditate on our inevitable death, get acquainted with it, evaluate it, argue with it, and get rid of dreadful early life deceptions surrounding it. We all share the pain of finitude, as well as the agony caused by this squirming fear at the core of our being. Now is an excellent time to dismiss the fallacy that passing away is too painful to endure, that reflection on it will devastate us, that impermanence should be renounced, lest reality make existence futile. Encountering death with the assistance of philosophy not only overwhelms the fear of it, but makes life more moving, more cherished, and livelier. I am hopeful that by embracing our human finiteness we will come to enjoy the greatness of each moment, the pleasure of plain existence, and boost our compassion both for ourselves and others.

The core Epicurean therapeutic argument is straightforward and easy to conceive. It goes like this: the fear of death is both alien to our nature and unjustifiable to our intellect. It rests on the false belief that the dead are capable of experiencing the loss of their life, and therefore are aware of being deprived of all the good things of life they would have enjoyed if they still lived. This justification conflicts with common sense considering that to be subjected to loss, one must exist prior to and after that loss, and we recognize that the dead cease to exist. Therefore, the fear of death can be treated by the mediation of the Epicurean philosophy claiming that death is irrelevant both to the living and the dead. The assimilation of this cutting-edge relief will tame the fear of death, free our life from the authority of fear, and introduce in its place the guidelines of pleasure-pain. That single restructuring of our belief system is sufficient to ameliorate the quality of our life, ensuring health and peace of mind.

I hope that with the help of the philosophy of Epicurus, you too will come to terms with your finitude and cope with the fear of it.

"Note to readers: The italicized sentences within the text correspond to the references at the end of each chapter."

Haris Dimitriadis
July 2019

A PERSONAL NOTE

Dear reader,

In my late sixties, I feel now—more pressing than ever—the need to come face to face with the prospect of my own death. In doing so I found comfort in researching the lifelong question of human mortality and sharing the findings with you. There were, of course, additional motives that induced me in dealing with this unpleasant issue at this point in time. First of all, eventually I came to recognize that living a pleasant life is intertwined with coming to terms with the fear of death. I found myself worried and even panicked when I was undergoing precautionary medicals tests and anticipated the worst outcomes at the appearance of the slightest illness. This negative thinking was reinforced by the experience of friends and relatives of a similar age or even younger passing away from terminal illnesses.

On top of this, my recent experience with a close relative of mine suffering from a terminal illness was the last straw. The successive outbreaks of his sufferings functioned as constant reminders of my own mortality and the pain of dying. His unfortunate handling of his approaching death struck me as an example to be avoided. By altogether denying the possibility of his death, he was not only intensifying his pain, but also placing a heavy burden on his loved ones. He was becoming fearful, demanding, and tiresome. He never reconciled himself with the idea of his death. He never gave up hope and fought for his life to the last stage, keeping away from any serious reflection on the prospect of his death. How upsetting, I thought, to have not been acquainted with and prepared for the inevitability of our own passing. How depressing to depart life shaken and disappointed. What a miserable legacy to bestow on our loved ones. I felt terrified visualizing myself behaving like this on my own deathbed. An intense desire and strong will swamped my existence to shield myself from the terror of death; to be able to relinquish life proudly and bravely; to bid farewell the world by voicing, "I have lived, it's time to go."

Despite being acquainted with the philosophy of Epicurus for almost 20 years now, I have so far unconsciously denied paying a serious consideration of my own death. Nonetheless, I came to realize that the fear of it lies covert, underneath every inch of my existence, undermining the quality of my life. I feel that as I am currently healthy and sane, now is the right time to come to terms with my finitude, both calmly and thoughtfully.

Dear reader, as Epicurus claimed, the art of living well and dying well is one and the same. It is never too early or too late to embrace philosophy in living happily and healing the fear of mortality.

Haris Dimitriadis
June 2019

CONTENTS

CHAPTER 1

OVERVIEW

"A right understanding that death is nothing to us makes the mortality of life enjoyable, not because it adds to it an infinite span of time, but because it takes away the craving for immortality. For there is nothing terrible in life for the man who has truly comprehended that there is nothing terrible in not living."

—Epicurus, *Letter to Menoeceus*

These days we are accustomed thinking of philosophy as an academic discipline studied in university and that to be a philosopher is to be a scholar of philosophy. But that is not always how it has been. Indeed, in ancient times it was in every respect conceivable to be a philosopher without having written a single word, for what was important was not being acquainted with philosophical theories, but living philosophically. Why do we have such a conflicting understanding of philosophy as an academic branch of knowledge today? The reason is that with the establishment of Christianity in the West as the sole religion of the states, there was no purpose in having philosophical schools to strive against each other, all claiming knowledge of the unique truth. If religion was the origin of truth about how to live our lives, then the task of philosophy would be of little importance. Its function would be to justify the tenets of religion, in view of the fact that it was religion itself – and not philosophy – that was the guide to life. In the present day, however, with the advance of pragmatism and the end of the sovereignty of theology, philosophy as a way of life can manifest itself once more, and there is no doubt that we see it again as having a strong say on how we live our lives.

The fear of death has been tormenting man since antiquity. Early philosophers, especially Epicurus, regarded this pervasive fear as the root cause of human misery; that is why he recognized the mental and ethical liberation of man from the chains of the fear of death as the supreme focus of his philosophy. Ever since man emancipated himself from the gods of myth and the imperative of fate, he has come to face a last necessity, the most inevitable of all: that of death. His release from the fear of death would be the ultimate achievement of Epicurus, supporting the belief that there is nothing terrible in life for anyone who understands that nothing terrible exists when he ceases to live. However, the course of events reversed his expectations. New religions emerged that promised the hope of immortality. They devised an afterlife, the resurrection, eternal joy, and feeling disappointed and desperate by the misery of everyday life, man embraced those words of relief despite having a deep suspicion that all these teachings were a delightful illusion.

On top of that, the emergence of the contemporary consumerist philosophy gave rise to a new cause of fear of death. This is based on the *idea of deprivation,* according to which death harms the dead in the form of defeated desires, undermined interests, and unfulfilled prospects. Epicurus argues that to make such declarations about death is senseless, since something must exist for it to be the subject of harm. Since the dead cannot be harmed, they evidently cannot be aggrieved by being deprived of anything. Harm is pain that is either physical or psychical and is perceived only through sense experience. Hence the phrase, *bad for one's life*, means only that one experiences pain before death. Moreover, for Epicurus, it is not the accomplishment of aspirations and tasks that convey meaning to life, but rather the pleasure of engaging in activities we like and enjoy. The Epicurean can enjoy full happiness in the moment, irrespective of successes or disappointments due to luck or need. What is really at issue in this dispute is not so much the right stance toward death but the right stance toward life.

The alarming picture of inescapable death affects our ability to appreciate life and leaves no joy untroubled. *Children at an early age* cannot help but note the flashes of impermanency around them—dead animals and pets, vanishing relatives, lamenting parents, packed cemeteries. Children often simply observe, wonder, and remain silent. Whenever they openly express their anxiety, their parents strive to find reassuring words or postpone the whole issue into the remote future or relieve children's fearfulness with death-rejecting myths of everlasting life, paradise, awakening, and reunion. The fear of death usually goes covert until adolescence. *Teenagers often become obsessed with death*; a few consider suicide; most play violent video games; others enjoy death-inspired songs or horror films; a few provoke death by taking reckless risks; the majority strives for a career and gets ahead with a family. Later, as children leave home and professional life peaks, the midlife crisis can occur and an uneasiness about death once again rears its head. From that stage on, worries about mortality are never far away from the mind. Denial of death and belief in eternal life reemerge as the conventional solutions to the reappearance of this anxiety.

In today's world, a corrosive denial of anything pertaining to death dominates—death has grown savage, a taboo detrimental to life. While we may suppose this reaction is instinctive, it is flawed. *Within the course of years,* death has been reformed from an undisputed event of Nature to something that can be prevented or circumnavigated, something that will not actually happen to us. Passing away at present is in many ways more appalling, more lonesome, automated, and dehumanized; at times it is even hard to make out technically when the moment of death has taken place. Dying becomes gloomy and detached because the patient is often taken out of his or her intimate habitat and dashed to an emergency ward. When a patient is seriously ill, he is often regarded like a person with no right to an opinion. It is society that decides if, when and where a patient should be treated. Death is removed from the hands of the dying and placed under the jurisdiction of the loved ones and the supervision of society. Under this social control, death is silently wiped out in order to preserve the serenity of society. For the sake of society, we must shun the unbearable emotion prompted by the repulsiveness of death and its presence in our otherwise happy lives. However, we should never neglect that the patient also has feelings, desires, and opinions and has the right to be heard.

While we ceaselessly adhere to our denial of death, in reality our life is not as a result improved; moreover, we cannot preserve denial forever; we cannot continuously and successfully pretend that we are safe; we can never completely defeat death anxiety—it is always there, keeping out of sight in some hidden recess of the mind. Epicurus insisted that the intimidating thought of inevitable death interferes with our enjoyment of life and leaves no pleasure undisturbed. He turns down the idea of denial and puts forward the idea that by genuinely facing our death, our chances blossom and we can become healthier, stronger, and more cheerful. He advises that as long as we cannot deny death, it is worth making an effort to take sovereignty of the fear of it.

References

"Letter to Menoeceus": See annex 3

"idea of deprivation": 1. Nussbaum, M C (1994). *The Therapy of Desire: Theory and Practice in Hellenistic Ethics.* Princeton. 2. Nagel, T (1979). *Death.* In Mortal Questions, 1-10. Cambridge: Cambridge University Press. 3. Pitcher, G (1984). *The Misfortunes of the Dead.* American Philosophical Quarterly 21(2): 183-88. 4. Feinberg, G (1984). *Harm to Others.* Oxford: Oxford University Press. Reprinted in part in Fischer. 5. Luper-Foy, S (1987). *Annihilation.* Philosophical Quarterly 37(148):233-252. Reprinted in Fischer. 6. Feldman, F (1991). *Some Puzzles about the Harm of Death.* Philosophical Review 100(2):205-27.

"bad for one's life": 1. Rosenbaum, Stephen E (1986). *How to Be Dead and Not Care: A Defense of Epicurus.* American Philosophical Quarterly, Vol. 23, No. 2 (Apr.) *2.* Mitsis, Phillip (2002). *Happiness and Death in Epicurean Ethics.* New York.

"Children at an early age": Yalom, Irvin (2011). *Staring at the Sun: Being at peace with your own mortality.* Piatkus; reprint edition.

"Teenagers often become obsessed with death": 1. Yalom, Irvin (2011). *Staring at the Sun: Being at peace with your own mortality.* 2. Nelli L Mitchell, and Karen R Schulman (1980). *The child and the fear of death.* Rochester, New York. 3. Karen Young. *Fear and Anxiety: An Age by Age Guide to Common Fears: The Reasons for Each and How to Manage Them.*

"Within the course of years": Philippe Ariès (1975). *Western Attitudes toward Death: From the Middle Ages to the Present (The Johns Hopkins Symposia in Comparative History).* Translated by Patricia Ranum.

Chapter 2

THE NATURE OF DEATH

"When the whole body is broken up, the soul is scattered and has no longer the same powers as before, nor the same notions; hence it does not possess sentience either."

—Epicurus, *Letter to Herodotus*

To avoid misconceptions, it is worthwhile clarifying that throughout this monograph we understand death to imply what Epicurus himself assumed to be: that it is the state of being dead. Epicurus is concerned neither with the process of dying or with any special feature of death, such as whether it is untimely, or cruel, or painful. He is interested simply in the loss of life, with the reality that we must pass away and be no more. For Epicurus, the correct understanding of death implies the ultimate end of life—death is not harmful to the dead; the features surrounding death are irrelevant to the dead; the harmful consequences of death are experienced by the loved ones and society; harmful is the pain endured in the process of dying. In other words, for Epicurus, the features surrounding death are not a subject matter entitled under the question of death, but under that of life. For example, whether a death is caused by torture over many hours versus dying peacefully in one's sleep is not an issue of interest to the dead but to the living. In front of a similar dilemma, Epicurus would ask: is it worthwhile suffering a long-lasting incurable illness or putting an end to our life on our own? Obviously, this decision has to do with life and the living and is of no concern to those that are already dead.

When most people visualize their death, they conceive themselves into a future self that experiences endless muted obscurity. However, this is fallacious because without sensation, there is no comprehension of space and time. Consciousness is all we are and all that we have: as far as we are concerned, being deprived of consciousness and our own self means that the entire world disintegrates into nothing-ness.

According to neuroscience, many proofs establish that the mind is of organic substance, functioning according to natural processes. If, for example, you send an electric current through a specific structure in the brain, you cause the person to have a vivid experience. If a part of the brain dies because of a blood clot or a burst artery or some other trauma, a part of the person is gone. An individual may lose the ability to see, think, or feel, and their entire personality may change. The same happens gradually when the brain accumulates a protein called beta-amyloid in the tragic disease of Alzheimer's. *The soul, which is the emotional circuitry of* the *brain*, gradually disappears as the brain decays from this physical process. We know that every form of intellectual activity, every emotion, every thought, and every conception emit electrical, magnetic, or metabolic signals that can be recorded with high accuracy by imaging techniques, such positron-emission tomography (PET) or magnetic resonance imaging (MRI). We know that if you look at the brain under a microscope, it has an astonishing degree of elaboration in the order of a trillion synapses, corresponding to the thrilling perplexity of human thought and experience. We know that when the brain dies, the person goes out of existence.

In physics, death is comparable to permanent oblivion; namely, there is no life after death. We each have a limited time as living beings and when it's over, it's over. If the atoms are what constitute each living organism, without any incorporeal soul, then the particulars that make up us are included in the alignment of atoms that constitute our body, including our brain. There is no location for that information to go or any way for it to be kept outside our body.

In philosophy, there are fundamentally two perspectives on death. The first is that it is a departure of the soul or consciousness from this world into another and that the souls of all perished people will also be in that domain. The other outlook on death is that it is the end, the absolute termination of consciousness, and leaves the individual not only incapable of feeling, but with a total absence of awareness, like a person in a deep and dreamless sleep.

The first thing that Epicurus strove to establish was the complete and permanent loss of consciousness at death. In order to comprehend the Epicurean view of the nature of death, it is essential to gain an understanding of the nature of the soul-body relationship because it forms the basis of establishing the irrationality of our fears concerning our own death. The human body is composed of the body and the mind, both of which have a physical reality. They are born together; they coexist throughout our lifetime. We cannot physically separate one from the other. They reflect different properties of the same thing. Therefore, once the entire body is dispersed along with the soul, as happens in death, the soul will have lost its powers of sense perception and motion. It is impossible in this case even to imagine the soul with its customary powers in a lifeless body.

Finally, the use of the term 'incorporeal' is valid only insofar as it refers to the void, for only the void can be conceived of as independently existing. And the void can neither act nor be acted upon but merely provides the possibility of motion through itself for bodies. Thus, it is an utter misconception *to regard the soul as incorporeal* as this would rob it of its essential characteristics, namely the ability to perceive and to act and be acted upon. Body and soul are material entities, so integrated as to account for the salient features of living men, intentions, perceptions, and actions, yet subject—like all atomic structures in the universe—to a dissolution that constitutes the death of these same creatures; and what has been dissolved has no sense experience, and what has no sense experience is nothingness. Therefore, Epicurus claims, death—which appears to be the most frightening of very bad things—should be nothing to us, since when we exist, death is not yet present, and when death is present, we do not exist. In other words, while we live we would be foolish indeed to dwell upon death and thereby allow it to prevent our living a good life. Our longing for immortality needs to be removed and we should prepare ourselves mentally for death, so that when that time comes, we will die without panic knowing that we have enjoyed life and will no longer have any sensation. This is because all good and bad relates to sense experience, and death is the end of sense experience. Hence, a correct understanding of the fact that death is nothing to us makes the mortality of life a matter of contentment, not by adding a limitless time to life, but by removing the longing for immortality.

While challenging and *furtively pushing death out* of the world of familiar things may feel like a permanent trait of humanity, historical research indicates that we have not always rejected our mortality as we do now. The attitude of the contemporary *man has not been sincere.* He resists that each and every person owes Nature his death and he must prepare himself to pay that debt—in short, that death is natural, unquestionable, and fatal. To rephrase it in the words of Epicurus, one can attain security against other things, but when it comes to death, all men live in a city without walls. We should never lose sight of the fact that we are animals and we should accept that our mortality as inescapable. On the ground of the pleasure-seeking philosophy of life, a good life can equal that of the gods, not in duration, but in fullness; and if to be immortal is to live without thinking of death, then the Epicurean sage is certainly immortal. Death is nothing to him. Absolutely nothing.

References

"Letter to Herodotus": See annex 4.

"to regard the soul as incorporeal": Epicurus, *letter to Herodotus.*

"The soul, which is the emotional circuitry of the brain": 1. LeDoux, J E (1996). *The Emotional Brain.* New York: Simon and Schuster Paperbacks. 2. LeDoux, J E 1998). *Fear and the brain: Where have we been, and where are we going? Biol.* Psychiatr. 1998; 44:1229–38. [PubMed] 3. LeDoux, J E (2000). *Emotion circuits in the brain.* Annu. Rev. Neurosci. 2000; 23:155–84. [PubMed]. 4. LeDoux, J E (2003). *Synaptic Self: How Our Brains Become Who We Are.* 5. LeDoux, J E (2019). *The Deep History of Ourselves: The Four-Billion-Year Story of How We Got Conscious Brains.* 6. Damasio, A (1994). *Descartes' Error: Emotion, Reason, and the Human Brain.* New York: Putnam's Sons. Revised Penguin edition, 2005. 7. Damasio, A 1999). *The Feeling of What Happens: Body and Emotion in the Making of Consciousness.* Harcourt. 8. Damasio, A (2003). *Looking for Spinoza: Joy, Sorrow, and the Feeling Brain.* Harcourt. 9. Damasio, A 2010). *Self Comes to Mind: Constructing the Conscious Brain.* Pantheon. 10. Damasio, A (2018). *The Strange Order of Things: Life, Feeling, and the Making of Cultures.* Pantheon.

"furtively pushing death out": Ariès, Philippe (1975). *Western Attitudes toward Death: From the Middle Ages to the Present* (The Johns Hopkins Symposia in Comparative History).

"man has not been sincere": Freud, Sigmund (1918). *Reflections on War and Death.*

CHAPTER 3

THE FEAR OF DEATH

"The man speaks but idly who says that he fears death not because it will be painful when it comes, but because it is painful in anticipation."

—Epicurus, *Letter to Menoeceus*

Epicurus considered the fear of death more detrimental to peace of mind than all other fears, except that of the fear of the gods. He used to say that men fear death in the same way that children fear to go into the dark and as fear in children is increased with tales, so it is the case for men. For some people, death anxiety is just *the background music of life*, and for others, a preoccupation with death can take dramatic forms. One imagines himself sealed in a coffin, covered with soil, yet sentient of being in darkness the entire time. Another dreads never seeing, hearing, or touching a loved one again. Others feel the sadness of being under the soil while friends are above it, unable of ever knowing what will happen to their family, friends, or the world. In many people, death anxiety is undisguised and easily identifiable, however heartbreaking that might be. In others it is hidden, and it is detected only by disciplined investigation. The emotions associated with death anxiety extend from a few fleeting instants of fear to a paralyzing condition of panic. In either case, the person is hurting or frightened. This is exactly why people prefer to minimize even their *cognitive encounters with death* and maintain a fantasy or illusion of immortality.

Death anxiety is a fear underlying numerous psychological conditions. *A large body of research* has been dedicated to the study of death anxiety and a number of consistent findings have emerged. In particular, *women typically report* higher death anxiety than men; higher education and socioeconomic status are moderately associated with lower death anxiety; older people do not typically report higher death anxiety than younger people; *religious beliefs and practices* are not necessarily associated with lower death anxiety; good physical health is associated with lower death anxiety; and more psychological problems are associated with higher levels of death anxiety. *There is considerable evidence* that end-of-life conditions may be associated with death anxiety, depression, and psychological distress. *There is also evidence* to suggest that higher death anxiety in end-of-life care is associated with higher prevalence and severity of psychiatric disorders such as generalized anxiety disorder (GAD) and depression. *Based on this evidence*, reducing psychological distress and death anxiety is a fundamental component of end-of-life care and treatment and has been associated with several psychosocial improvements, such as a reduction in depression and anxiety, enhanced quality of life, decreased pain, and improved coping skills.

Both theoretical knowledge and clinical observation suggest that the sense of threat experienced in disorders such as *hypochondriasis and health anxiety* is related to a pathological fear of death. This fear has also been disclosed by patients with *medically unexplained symptoms*, highlighting the potential for death anxiety to run across many somatic symptoms and related disorders. Indeed, *there is evidence to suggest that the fear of death* is a universal factor underlying all phobias. For example, many obsessive-compulsive tendencies are significantly linked with mortality-related concerns about the self or loved ones, while reminders of death are intensifying compulsive behaviors. This suggests that mortality salience—i.e. the ability to recognize and accept an impending death—may be a general factor in the experience of obsessive-compulsive disorder and may in some way explain the exaggerated focus that individuals with obsessive-compulsive issues place on the elimination of germs, disease, and danger. For example, someone with a phobia of spiders may feel that they are threatening when they actually pose no harm. This would make more sense if the spider phobic experienced a reminder of death even when the spider is not deadly. That is, *the exaggerated nature of phobic fears* may be triggered or exacerbated by an underlying fear of death. Besides, *several agoraphobic symptoms and fears* are associated with a fear of death, including fear of anticipated harm and death-related catastrophes. *Depressive disorders may be* also associated with or exacerbated by existential despair and lack of meaning.

Why do we fear death? *Self-awareness is a supreme gift*, a treasure as precious as life itself. This is what makes us human, but it comes at a costly price: the wound of mortality. Our existence is forever shadowed by the knowledge that we will grow, blossom, and inevitably diminish and die. When facing danger, our consciousness perceives and evaluates the risk involved to protect our lives, enhancing the possibility of our survival. This capacity of the mind carries with it the realization that our very nature is vulnerable, limited, and mundane, and it raises feelings of terror and persistent thoughts focused on avoiding our inevitable death. Ever since, a fear of death has become covert and unconsciously influences almost all of our activities. *On the positive side,* self-awareness of mortality offers an opportunity for authentic existence and an appreciation of life. It serves as motivation to pursue potential and create an uplifting sense of joy; yet additionally it can fill an individual with a concurrent realization that all things must come to an end. We become aware of the fact that this is the only life available to us and we should enjoy its pleasures and delights without delay. Regrettably, many people are preoccupied with the idea, and even the dread, of impermanence. What's the point in anything, they ask, if everything will eventually die away? Each and every enjoyable activity is transitory and may end at any moment. Any pleasant feeling is doomed to vanish like all the other splendid things in life. Of course, no one could question the ephemerality of all things and also question the view that the transience of what is fascinating increases rather than decreases its value. Epicurus used to say that just as one does not unconditionally choose the largest amount of food but the most pleasant food, he savors not the longest time, but the most pleasant.

A major source of death anxiety is existential in nature, which stems from the basic knowledge that human life must end. Many people fear the idea that they will entirely cease to exist after death happens. This is the fear of death as personal annihilation, *the fear of going to the underworld* is matched with the fear of going nowhere. Some are swayed by the immensity of eternity, of being dead forever and ever; others are unable to take hold of the state of nonbeing and ask the question of where they will be when they are dead; others struggle with the notion of the fatality of death. The reality is that death can never be fully understood by anyone who is living since no one in human history has survived it to tell us what really happens after we take our last breath. Death continues to be the terminal mystery of human beings throughout time. *A related existential view of death* proposes that the human motivation to stay alive, coupled with the awareness that death can occur at any time, has the power to engender paralyzing fear of it; to manage or tranquilize this existential fear of death, *people employ cultural worldviews and self-esteem* as an anxiety-buffering shield.

Intense experiences, both positive and negative, also trigger existential dread. Negative experiences, such as failure to achieve an important life goal or a painful personal rejection, can bring to light covert death fears. Likewise, a loss or ending, casualties, symptoms of aging, ill health, and subjection to risk often upset a person's sense of confidence and security prompting the mind to make symbolic associations of them with death and dying. At the same time, positive experiences, such as a major achievement or recognition, falling in love and making a commitment in a relationship, may initiate feelings of fear in recognition of the prospect that although life is precious, it must eventually be surrendered. Equally, pleasant experiences such as birthdays and holidays make us mindful of time passing and arouse covert feelings of mortality salience.

Many people fear an eternal punishment in Hell for what they did or did not do while on Earth. They might find comfort in religion, which introduces a belief system based on the existence of some form of life after death. God pledges to the faithful to palliate their suffering of the impermanence of life, but also to alleviate the dreadful solitude of the afterlife. *For the Epicurean* philosopher-poet, such fears are unfounded as it is in this life that men are so oppressed by their own unbridled worries that they live as if in Hell. Torments that are said to take place in the depths of Hell are actually present now in our own lives.

A popular cause of fear of death stems from the idea of deprivation based on the delusion that death deprives dead people of certain goods he or she would have enjoyed if they had not died. This reasoning is based on the unfairness of premature death by submitting that unexpected death prevents the deceased from enjoying all the goods he has acquired through struggle and sacrifice during his life. It goes on by presenting the following example: *consider two lives,* one very short and cut off prematurely and the other fully provided, containing enjoyment to a ripe old age. Isn't it obvious, they ask, that the second life is to be thought of as better than the first? Others raise a similar argument in support of the notion of the unlived life, which refers to the terror and nightmares caused by our sense that time is running out and our life is slipping away. In line with this rationale, the more unlived your life, the greater your death anxiety. The more you fail to experience your life fully, the more you will fear death. On the other hand, some bring forward a counter argument in support of the view that it is the loss of our past that frightens us most. They maintain that we carry with us all the memories of our experiences, preferences, desires, the presence of our loved ones, and all of our possessions. How devastating to reconcile with the idea that we are doomed to desert all of them? If we were in absolute isolation, we would probably renounce them with less difficulty.

Similar statements make no sense, since they disregard the simple truth that the end is not capable of being experienced and consequently the particulars of death are irrelevant to the dead, no matter what they are. Comparisons are meaningful only between the living beings, not between the dead or a living being and a dead body. Death is neither evil nor good to the dead. It is nothingness.

Another source of death anxiety is related to *standing out and being different.* Whenever we move out of the familiar safety of social consensus and expand our lives, anxiety is aroused or heightened. By becoming aware of our separateness, we begin to experience aloneness, vulnerability, and fear of mortality. Similarly, taking critical decisions for personal growth, relinquishing dependency ties, separating from illusions of connection, and moving toward a more independent attitude in life causes anxiety and can activate fears of dying. A familiar example is differentiating from parental and societal binds, which brings forth unconscious death fears in anticipation of being rejected by family or society.

Similarly, the perception of losing control in confronting death alarms a large number of people and causes panic attacks and distress. While generally we are fond of being in charge of the circumstances we come across, coping with death is embarrassing and frightening since our only knowledge or experience of it is entirely theoretical or at most, indirectly learned through the death of others. On top of that, negative thinking accentuates the feeling of distress by envisaging the pain and suffering that accompanies the dying process. The usual reaction to these fears is to become exceedingly cautious or go through meticulous, recurring health checkups.

Many people are not virtually as afraid to die as they are of what would happen to their loved ones after their death. They may be anxious that their friends and family would have a bad time financially or that no one would be around to support them. Others are not so fearful of their own death, but the death of a loved one. They are terrified by the possibility of the death of a parent, a wife or husband, a brother or sister, a child, or a dear friend.

As mentioned earlier, the idea of death and the recognition of a limited existence develops progressively as a child grows up. *Young children get familiar* with the reality of death when a pet dies or when an elderly relative passes away. Gradually children learn that their mother and father are also susceptible to death. Soon they come to understand that they too cannot sustain their own lives forever. From this moment on, the dread of death is unbearable and is inevitably repressed. Even though defense mechanisms keep it away from consciousness, children's fears are saved in their totality in the unconscious memory. Continual-ly, the suppressed fear of death keeps on exercising an intense grip on the life of the child and later the adult.

The fear of death also has positive effects on our life. Just as physical pain motivates us to refrain from bodily harm, so fear of death stimulates sensible and watchful behavior to support our self-preservation and make the most of our time here on Earth. On top of that, it can result in *positive changes* such as a greater appreciation for life, a shift in priorities toward intrinsic goals, and improved interpersonal relationships. In other words, we are moved to reassess our values, readjust our preferences, avoid the things we do not enjoy, and embrace the pleasure of companionship and the simple joys of life.

Despite its universality, the fear of death is not intrinsic to human nature. The child has no awareness of death until between the ages of three to five. It is too intangible an idea, too alien to his life. He enjoys himself in a reality that is full of feeding, playing, entertaining, and acting. He is ignorant of what it means for life to vanish, nor is he capable of speculating where it would go. Only little by little does he learn that there is death that takes people away forever; very hesitantly comes to accept that it sooner or later, it takes everyone away, but this step by step comprehension of the certainty of death can take up until puberty.

Mankind does have *organic fears* ingrained in the unconscious such as a fear of altitude, darkness, loud noises, and certain animals. In those hidden places of our mind there is no trace of information about death. *The unconscious is not occupied with death* since it is not something that it has come into contact with. We know that repeated exposure over a long period of time becomes coded gradually into our genes. Nonetheless, death is not an experience of a living human being and naturally there is no way for it to turn into an innate feature of our brain. Basically, in the unconscious every one of us is persuaded of his own deathlessness. The fear of death, which manipulates us all the time, is subordinate and the result of mindfulness.

An additional argument in support of this claim can be drawn by observing how primitive people lived their life. Those people reflected a little and were occupied with no more than pleasure, where enjoyment was the supreme good, and where food and water were the most enjoyable things. They had little or no fear of death, and often they challenged it fearlessly. Does this behavior of the primitive people not prove that the fear of death is not an organic feature of the human mind? A similar conclusion emerges by watching the behavior of animals. Isn't it striking that they are completely unaware of death?

For Epicurus, there are no good reasons to look at the fear of death as rational either. On the contrary, there are many accounts for asserting such a fear to be – in all respects – irrational. The following four-step syllogism is a straightforward proof of this: 1. An event can be good or bad for someone only if, at the time when the event is present, that person exists as a subject, so that it is at least possible that the person experiences the event; 2. The time after a person dies is a time at which that person does not exist as a subject of possible experience, hence the condition of being dead is not bad for that person; 3. It is irrational to fear a future event unless that event, when it comes, will be bad for one; 4. Conclusion: it is irrational to fear death .

The words 'loss' or 'deprivation' appear to be at the heart of the contemporary fear of death. Nonetheless, utilizing these words in regards to death arguments is mistaken because for someone to be subject to a loss, he must exist both before and after the loss. Otherwise, the word 'loss' is self-contradicting and meaningless. We may suspect then, that the idea of deprivation rests upon the false cultural belief that the dead are not quite dead, but rather they hold on to some sort of life after their demise. For this reason, Epicurus rightly renounces the fear of death and asserts that one can overcome it by the mediation of philosophy. The preferred attitude is to be indifferent to death and be engrossed in enjoying ourselves for as long as we live. To put it differently, instead of being negatively motivated by fear, we should be positively motivated by pleasure. That simple transformation of perspective will stimulate a dramatic boost in our psychology and improve the quality of our life.

The wise man is scared neither to live or to die, and he will care not about living the longest life, but rather *the most pleasant one*. In fact, Epicurus says the same pattern of being leads to a good life and a good death. Death as complete extinction is the outcome of the Epicurean analysis considering the soul as a temporary amalgam of atomic particles. *The moral corollary of it* is that we should not let the fear of death ruin our life. Hopefully, in spite of the continuous presence of this fear in our lives, the natural human drive for survival and happiness still endures. Just let's look at how children indulge in playing; how absorbed they are in their activities; how intensely they enjoy the flow of the moment. In turn, *adults are so occupied with* pursuing a family, raising children, chasing their ambitions, and enjoying their lives, that the idea of death rarely crosses their minds. The urge to live happily is apparent in all human actions even when the outlook of our life shrinks and clouds over.

References

"the background music of life": Yalom, Irvin (2011). *Staring at the Sun: Being at peace with your own mortality.*

"Death anxiety is a fear underlying": 1. Arndt, J, Routledge, C, Cox, C R, & Goldenberg, J L (2005). *The worm at the core: A terror management perspective on the roots of psychological dysfunction.* Applied and Preventive Psychology, 11. 2. Furer, P, & Walker, J R (2008). *Death anxiety: A cognitive–behavioral approach.* Journal of Cognitive Psychotherapy, 22. 3. Strachan, E, Schimel, J, et al. (2007). *Terror mismanagement: Evidence that mortality salience exacerbates phobic and compulsive behaviors.* Personality and Social Psychology Bulletin, 33, 1137–1151.

"cognitive encounters with death": Kastenbaum, Robert (2000). *The psychology of death (3rd ed.).* New York: Springer Publishing.

"A large body of research": 1. Clinical Psychology Review (2014). *Death anxiety and its role in psychopathology: Reviewing the status of a transdiagnostic construct,* Volume 34, Issue 7, November 2014. 2. Furer, P, and Walker, John R (2008). *Death Anxiety: A Cognitive-Behavioral Approach.* Journal of Cognitive Psychotherapy: An International Quarterly, Volume 22, Number 2.

"women typically report": Wass, H, Berardo, F M, & Neimeyer, R A (1988). *Dying: Facing the facts.* 2nd ed. New York, NY, US: Hemisphere Publishing Corp/Harper & Row Publishers.

"religious beliefs and practices": 1. Ahmed MAbdel-Khalek (2009). *Religiosity and Subjective Well-being in the Arab Context.* 2. Jong, Jonathan, Halberstadt, Jamin (2016). *Death Anxiety and Religious Belief: An Existential Psychology of Religion.*

"There is considerable evidence": 1. Lagerdahl, A, Moynihan, M, and Stollery, B (2014). *An Exploration of the Existential Experiences of Patients Following Curative Treatment for Cancer* Journal of Psychosocial Oncology, Volume 32, 2014, Issue 5. 2. Royal, K D, and Elahi, F (2011*). Psychometric properties of the Death Anxiety Scale (DAS) among terminally ill cancer patients. Journal of Psychosocial Oncology, 29, 359– 371.* 3. Spiegel, D (1995). *Essentials of psychotherapy intervention for cancer patients. Supportive Care in Cancer, 3, 252–256.*

"There is also evidence": Krause, S, Rydall, A, Hales, S, Rodin, G, & Lo, C (2014). *Initial validation of the Death and Dying Distress Scale for the assessment of death anxiety in patients with advanced cancer.* Journal of Pain and Symptom Management.

"Based on this evidence": 1*.* Menzies, Rachel and Menzies, Ross (2018). *Curing the Dread of Death: Theory, Research and Practice.* 2. Lo, C, Hales, et al. (2011). *Measuring death-related anxiety in advanced cancer: Preliminary psychometrics of the Death and Dying Distress Scale.* Journal of Pediatric Hematology and Oncology, 33, S140eS145. 3. Lo, C, Hales, et al. (2014). *Managing Cancer and Living Meaningfully (CALM): Phase 2 trial of a brief individual psychotherapy for patients with advanced cancer.* Palliative Medicine. 4. Sherman, D W, Norman, R, & McSherry, C, B (2010). *A comparison of death anxiety and quality of life of patients with advanced cancer or AIDS and their family caregivers.* Journal of the Association of Nurses in AIDS Care, 21, 99–112.

"hypochondriasis and health anxiety": 1. Starcevic, Vladan and Noyes, Russell Jr. (2014). *Hypochondriasis and Health Anxiety: A guide for Clinicians.* 2. Furer, P, Walker, et al. (1997*). Hypochondriacal concerns and somatization in panic disorder.*

Depression and Anxiety, 6, 78–85. 3. Furer, P, Walker, J R, & Stein, M B (2007). *Treating health anxiety and fear of death: A practitioner's guide for Clinicians.* New York: Springer Publishing.

"medically unexplained symptoms": Cowen, Philip, Paul Harrison. (2012). *Shorter Oxford Textbook of Psychiatry.*

"there is evidence to suggest that the fear of death": Kingman, R (1928). *Fears and phobias: Part II. Welfare Magazine, 19, 303–308.*

"the exaggerated nature of phobic fears": Strachan, E, Schimel, J, et al. (2007). *Terror mismanagement: Evidence that mortality salience exacerbates phobic and compulsive behaviors.* Personality and Social Psychology Bulletin, 33.

"several agoraphobic symptoms and fears": Starcevic, Vladan (2010). *Anxiety Disorders in Adult: A Clinical Guide.*

"Depressive disorders may be": 1. Simon, L, Arndt, et al. (1998). *Terror management and meaning: Evidence that the opportunity to defend the worldview in response to mortality salience increases the meaningfulness of life in the mildly depressed.* Journal of Personality, 66. 2. Stopa, Lusia (2009*). Imagery and the Threatened Self: Perspectives on Mental Imagery and the Self in Cognitive Therapy.*

"Self-awareness is a supreme gift": Yalom, Irvin (2011). *Staring at the Sun: Being at peace with your own mortality.*

"On the positive side": 1. Evans, C Stephen (2009). *Kierke-gaard: An Introduction.* 2. Heidegger, Martin (1962). *Being and Time.* Translated by Macquarrie, John & Robinson, Edward.

"the fear of going to the underworld": Seneca, *Letters from a Stoic, Epistulae Morales Ad Lucilium 82.16.* Translated By Robin Campbell, Penguin Books (1969).

"A related existential view of death": Becker, Ernest (1973). *The Denial of Death. Penguin ed. P. 88, lines 866–870.*

"people employ cultural worldviews and self-esteem": 1. Greenberg, J, Solomon, et al. (1992). *Assessing the terror management analysis of self-esteem: Converging evidence of an anxiety-buffering function.* Journal of Personality and Social Psychology, 63. 2. Hayes, J, Schimel, S, et al. (2010). *A theoretical and empirical review of the death-thought accessibility concept in terror management research.* Psychological Bulletin, 136. 3. Pyszczynski, T, Greenberg, J, & Solomon, S (1999). *A dual-process model of defense against conscious and unconscious death-related thoughts: An extension of terror management theory.* Psychological Review, 106. 4. Routledge, C (2012). *Failure causes fear: The effect of self-esteem threat on death anxiety.* Journal of Social Psychology, 152, 665–669. 5. Strachan, E, Schimel, et al. (2007). *Terror mismanagement: Evidence that mortality salience exacerbates phobic and compulsive behaviors.* Personality and Social Psychology Bulletin, 33, 1137–1151.

"For the Epicurean philosopher-poet": Lucretius. *On the Nature of things.* Translated by Cyril Bailey (1910). Oxford press.

"consider two lives": 1. Williams, Bernard (1973). *Problems of the Self.* Cambridge: Cambridge University Press. 2. Furley, D J (1986). *"Nothing to Us?"* In Schofield and Striker. 3. Long, A A, and Sedley, D (1987). *The Hellenistic Philosophers.* 2 vols. Cambridge.

"standing out and being different": Irvin D Yalom (1980). Existential Psychotherapy.

"Young children get familiar": Yalom, Irvin (2011). *Staring at the Sun: Being at peace with your own mortality.*

"positive changes": 1. Tedeschi, R G, & Calhoun, L G (1996). *The Posttraumatic Growth Inventory: Measuring the Positive Legacy of Trauma.* 2. Tedeschi, R G, & Calhoun, L G (2004). *Posttraumatic growth: Conceptual foundations and empirical evidence.* 3. Lykins, Emily, L, B, Segerstrom, et al. (2007). *Goal shifts following reminders of mortality: reconciling posttraumatic growth and terror management theory.*

"organic fears": LeDoux, Joseph (1998). 1. The emotional brain: The mysterious underpinnings of emotional life. 2. Sigmund Freud (1918). *Reflections on War and Death.*

"The unconscious is not occupied with death": Sigmund Freud (1918). *Reflections on War and Death.*

"the most pleasant one": Haris Dimitriadis (2017). *Epicurus and the Pleasant Life: A Philosophy of Nature.* 1st Edition.

"The moral corollary of it": Long, A A, and Sedley, D (1987). The Hellenistic Philosophers. 2 vols. Cambridge.

"adults are so occupied with": 1. Diener, Ed and Diener, Carol (1996). *Most People Are Happy.* Research Article. 2. *What keep us going:* Pew Research Center (2006). *Are we happy yet?*

CHAPTER 4

DEATH DENIAL: DEFENSES AGAINST DEATH ANXIETY

"Men are running away from themselves, filled with self-hatred, no one knowing what they really want and everyone is forever trying to get away from where he is, as though mere locomotion could throw off the load. The source of this anxious self-loathing turns out to be fear of the death that awaits all men."

—Lucretius, *On the Nature of Things*

The intelligence of men allows them to realize that they will someday die. This understanding brings about the stress of finitude. The most effective defense mechanisms for man to transcend the tragedy of their mortality include a symbolic form, such as living on in society and culture (perhaps as a famous author or for renowned wit and raconteur), and alternatively a literal sense of immortality that can be achieved through varying commitment to a religion. These immortality mechanisms are graded in four levels; the first and most fundamental level is the personal one. It is the level of the self-esteemed self, the gifted self, the heroic image of our own existence. The second level is the social; it impersonates the most cherished continuance of oneself to a select few exclusive others: a partner, friends, relatives, and conceivably even pets. The third level is the secular; it is composed of symbols of devotion further away from us and frequently more powerful, such as the company, the party, the country, and humanity. Lastly, the fourth and highest level is the sacred. It is the unseen, faceless level of power, for instance Nature or God.

Some of the defenses against death anxiety have favorable side effects; for example, projecting ourselves through creative works; discovering meaning in commitment to family, as well as in leaving a socially beneficial legacy. On the other hand, most defenses usually form the basis of multiple harmful actions as violation of rules, frantic rituals, and obsession over wealth and power. Along with these acts, mental issues manifest themselves in a variety of symptoms, *such as inner conflicts,* worries, stresses, depression, and even schizophrenia. Negation of our mortality brings about issues that may not at first seem directly connected to death. Often they are underground and are made known in signals that seem uncorrelated to mortality. In the short term they could be helpful by providing time to adjust to disturbing news, but excessive use of it is emotionally costly.

While we would expect that the awareness of our ultimate demise would discourage us from enjoying our lives, we nevertheless manage to cope with death anxiety by employing various defense mechanisms, such as creativity, raising children, boosting self-esteem, and accumulating wealth and power. While generally these mechanisms create a buffer against existential anxiety, several factors may *disable the effectiveness of them*, including genetic predispositions, adverse events in early childhood, temperament, insecure attachment, lack of meaning, trauma, stress, and other life difficulties. The inability to develop and use these essential components of the anxiety-buffering system is likely to result in psychological vulnerability and harm.

Defense through boosting self-esteem

Converging evidence supports the anxiety-buffer hypothesis that self-esteem is the primary buffer that serves to protect humans from death anxiety and to deny mortality. Growing a sense of personal significance and value increases the acceptance of threatening health messages and lessens worries of mortality by supporting an emblematic self that is more substantive than the everyday self. *To have feelings of self-worth* is to have a belief you are not just an animal destined to perish and be overlooked, but instead one who has lived a life of resolution and meaning and has made a powerful and surviving contribution to a meaningful and sustainable world. In this view, when individuals feel that they are meeting the specific standards of value *espoused by their culture*, they are provided with a sense of self-esteem that functions to buffer anxiety that in many cases is tethered to deeply rooted existential fears.

All civilizations advocate remedies of personal worth by way of divine or worldly processes. Whether one is struggling to be a rock star, a top athlete, a prolific scientist, a good citizen, or a dedicated member of the church, sustaining self-esteem is essential to being an authentic human. *People may be disposed of* for self-sacrifice to live up to cultural norms and values, for example they may be willing to die for their country unless an alternative means to affirm a transcendent self is offered. Others, instead of boosting self-esteem through authentic achievements, develop an inflated favorable opinion of themselves in order to counterbalance feelings of weakness and inadequacy and strengthen the sense of exemption from the destiny that is in store for all mankind. Few appear to be indifferent to a plain life, and as a consequence, exaggerate everyday problems by turning them into melodramas. They frequently behave with anger, fear, and panic over straightforward daily challenges, in order to be preoccupied over these less meaningful worries that are separate from death anxiety.

Defense through creativity

While one reason for creativity is that we see the world on our own terms and rely on ourselves to give meaning and eternity to our lives, another one is that a person needs *some kind of resolution* in a new and greater ideal, a freely chosen pursuit. Whether it is a work of art or literature, or perhaps an innovation, or a design that reflects the creator's persona and can last longer than the creator, the creative solution is a means to eternity. Through inspiration, we can convey our fleeting brevity onto our labor and be able to confront, appreciate, and address our finiteness through our achievement. *The current findings back up* the view that innovative accomplishment may be a boulevard for symbolic immortality, in particular among those who appreciate creativity. We are all going to pass away one day, but it becomes an event that's simpler to tolerate if you are leaving something worthwhile behind. Despite your body's ephemerality, indirectly some part of you will still be sticking around. Not only does creativity seem to shield people from mortality anxiety, but conversely, reminders of death also fuel creativity. For example, it is not surprising that many people have an increased need and desire for creativity when they are diagnosed with a terminal illness. It turns out that the concept of creation may be a beneficial mechanism to cope with the fear of death.

Defense through frenetic activity

A common defense mechanism to the fear of death is avoiding being alone and embracing a life of intense activity. People can find that they are running away from themselves, filled with self-hatred, no one knowing what they really want and everyone forever trying to get away from where he is, as though mere locomotion *could throw off the load*. The source of this anxious self-loathing turns out to be fear of the death that awaits all mankind. This is what initiates the escapist mania, and its consequences are ambition, greed, mistrust, and the running sores of life fed by fear of death. These practices not only fall short of extinguishing our thirst for immortality but end up in an aversion of life itself rather than an aversion for the end of life. In general, the zeal and obsession by which we pursue our activities can only be justified by the overwhelming feeling that our time on Earth is limited and running out.

Defense through accumulation of wealth, fame, and power

Some people compensate for their death fears by attempting to gain control over others and by achieving financial power. Research findings show that fear of death appears to be at the heart of people's propensity toward materialism and consumption. This attitude is associated with the free market culture recommending to individuals that *they are worthy members* of their culture to the degree that they have wealth, power, and fame. Indeed, money has more value than mere purchasing power. It carries with it both symbolic and emotional value that is capable of managing existential anxiety, particularly death anxiety. It provides one with a sense of control over life by acquiring things that help enhance health and safety. Although being in possession of some savings plays a psychological role as a buffer against death anxiety, it seems that having more money does not cause less anxiety. The wealthy may not lie awake at night worrying about paying their bills, but they do cringe when they hear reports that could topple their status of wealth. They could worry about interest rates or the stock market or if it is time to buy or sell real estate. The darker side of it, however, is that *the emphasis on wealth* is associated with poor well-being, stressful interpersonal relationships, and a lower quality of life. This is not to say that being wealthy, famous and powerful always results in a lower quality of life. Certainly, it can be used to fund pleasure, which can be construed as a good thing. Money, for example, can buy me and my loved ones holidays, good times, nice possessions, a healthy diet, excellent medical care, et cetera. Nonetheless, repeated research shows that, on average, few wealthy, famous, and powerful people are genuinely happy because the majority of them become exhausted or sick in the process of acquiring these 'goods', and as a result are unable to enjoy them.

Defense of living on through our children

Most people search for eternal life through their children. However, *children are only capable of* comforting or cushioning the death anxiety of their parents if they follow the lifestyle and convictions of them. Otherwise, if parents just want their children to be happy in their choices, the death anxiety of both parents and children is not eased. Many children have suffered in their development from their parents' efforts to make them into carbon copies of themselves. Children who feel they have to live up to their parent's dreams and ambitions will often try very hard initially because they want to please their parents, but for many of them, resentment, frustration, and even anger can set in, either as a child or when reflecting back on choices made as a young adult.

Defense through culture

The mortality salience hypothesis states that cultural worldviews provide a buffer from death anxiety, and that brushes with death, such as the serious illness of a loved one, will increase the need of individuals to strengthen their own worldview. Considering the psychological importance of denial of death, people tend to automatically surrender to what their culture prescribes as the right way to live. These individuals follow tradition unconditionally, do not ask questions, and robotically engage with their world. They come to believe that despite their bodily death, they will continue to live on through the immortality of society. Culture operates as a structure that scales down our tension about death by making provisions of symbolic immortality. The fundamental practice by which we run away from our death is the espousal and safety of our culture. Culture procures a remedy to our dread by giving us a new and durable life beyond that of the organic one. On top of that, in order to support our delusion that we will not in reality die, *we must disapprove and fight* all cultural schemes that seem likely to endanger and foreshadow the authority of our culture.

As a consequence, frequently this tendency to defend our ethnic character leads to mistreating others. If our cultural entity is endangered, then our essential feeling of deathlessness is imperiled and in an effort to keep escaping from death, we may end up wiping off any other conviction that challenges our own. We act as the champions who struggle with all those who pose a threat to our cultural identity. Our epic assignments at fighting vice have the seemingly absurd consequence of conveying more viciousness into the society. We justify ourselves in damaging others by imagining that those at variance to us are fundamentally and invariably ethically corrupt, extremists, or lunatics. In our hostility to the savage other, we are asserting our immortality by making the world more equitable, attractive, and friendly.

A defense mechanism related to culture is fetishizing specific cultural heroes. It doesn't matter whether *the cultural hero-system* is frankly magical, religious, primitive or secular, scientific, or civilized. It is still a mythical hero-system in which people serve in order to have a feeling of primary value, of cosmic importance, of ultimate usefulness to creation, and of unshakable meaning. Our connection to the immortal cosmos of the hero reflects on ourselves, allowing the assimilation of the superhuman qualities of the idol.

Defense through ritualistic behaviors

To avoid a direct confrontation with death and support a concept of immortality, man invented the theory of dualism, according to which humans are made up of a corporeal fatal body and a non-corporeal immortal soul. Even if the body vanishes, the soul survives death, and subsequently one need not fear death. That is the trick, but does it work? Clinical observations show that the majority of dying people find no escape from the terrors of death. *Even believing in a God* or an afterlife of any kind will not save us from the conflicts and fears of dying. Very few genuinely religious people with a deep-rooted faith were found to have been relieved by their beliefs and are best likened to those few who were true atheists. The preponderance of people nevertheless appear to continue to be restless and anxious at the thought of death.

Religion manipulated the concept of the dualistic nature of man to provide the hope of immortality. It preaches that by submitting yourself in the service of God, you have lived your life truly and wisely; by living with courage, resignation, dignity, and faith you certify your divine nature and compliance with God's will. You give your life its true completion, its genuine grandeur; God will make good use of your service whether it is good to you in any personal way, say, by way of spiritual immortality, or by way of being introduced into still secret dimensions of extraterrestrial life, in some kind of incarnation; or simply for the purpose of praise and embellishment of God himself. Curious as it may appear, while societies have been resorting increasingly to denial of death, less people believe in a life after death, and *religious mortality comfort has been diminishing*.

Mental symptoms of death denial

Negation of our mortality hinders us from taking hold of our possibilities and enjoying our lives to the full. The protective shield of society may be helpful in the short term, but evidence demonstrates that denying *the fatality of death* leads in the long run to anxiety. For some the symptoms are implicit, either as common anxiety or disguised as some other emotional syndrome. Few grow so fearful that they avoid activities with the slightest element of risk. Others suffer from a dramatic decline in work productivity. For some, the fear of death is conveyed through obsessive thoughts, nightmares, and panic. In particular, *studies show that patients* with panic disorder reported substantially greater anxiety about death than people without such disorders. They frequently fear they will faint, collapse, and die as a result of a panic attack. Others regularly consult with doctors regarding a *fear of dying from a heart attack*. In addition, many specific phobias are associated with a fear of objects or situations that carry the potential for harm or death, such as flying, ascending heights, confronting dangerous animals, and blood disorders. Research also suggests that death anxiety may be featured in the experience of *separation anxiety disorder and agoraphobia*. Inwardness is also a common mental disorder employed as a defense mechanism to retreat into ourselves to secure our independence and immortality. Introversion is basically a denial of engaging in society and is actualized as loneliness and self-care—by satisfying our wants and needs on our own and avoiding intimacy and involvement in emotional bonds, we create conditions of safety and immortality within our lonely world.

Similarly, several people adjust to death anxiety by having recourse to self-denial and withholding of affirmative feedback, talents, and potential, in order to keep them safe from others. In systematically disengaging from life, they get more detached from death; in a sense, they decline to wholly engage in a life they will definitely lose. To avoid the anguish of loss, they keep within their bounds or push aside loved ones by suppressing the attractive traits that their partner treasures in them. They get uneasy when they are intimately loved or cherished and react by positing restraints on the amount of love and devotion they are willing to offer and receive in a relationship, seeing that on the one hand, being loved makes them mindful of and contented with their lives, but on the other it makes them aware of the mere fact that they will ultimately lose those who love them.

Most forms of death denial require *opposition to others* in terms of the tyranny practiced within the society, and in terms of victimizing aliens or enemies outside it. Transferring our hostility onto someone else makes it possible to detach ourselves from our mortal existence, strengthen our identity within our immortal community, and divert our attention from the fear of our inevitable death. Of course there is no need for the adversary to be any race or even human being but it could also be an abstraction such as poverty, disability, or immigration. Furthermore, certain addictions—first and foremost food, drugs, and alcohol— directly or implicitly assist people in keeping a distance from death anxiety. Likewise, monotonous behaviors, routines, and obsessive work practices paralyze a person's susceptibility to negative feelings and provides an air of safety and immortality. *Obsessive thoughts and practice* ease death fears for a short time, but sooner or later they get accustomed and spark off even more anxiety. Furthermore, some people undertake small self-destructive acts day after day, with the intention of shirking from existential angst; in an effort to take a hold of their future, they waive elements of their lives in a series of self-denial and self-defeating attitudes. Moreover, there is evidence to suggest that non-effective suicidal attempts operate as a defensive disposition to death anxiety in a similar manner to a convict on death row who tries to end his life with the intention of keeping some control over his death, instead of tolerating the anxiety and agony in anticipation of his execution. Suicidal actions may range from abstinence to substance abuse, introversion, self-destructive attitude, self-inflicted injuries, and ritual suicide. These practices may at first seem incomprehensible, but *research has shown* that self-destructive or suicidal behaviors can act as a comfort and distraction to death anxiety.

A primary human incentive is denial of death. What we think, believe, do, and feel is motivated by our longing to avoid our departure from this life. In renouncing death, we may transfer ourselves into the future through our children; or we might become rich, famous, and powerful; we invent soothing practices, or introduce a belief in an ultimate rescuer. Some live heroically, often without taking into account the safety of others and themselves; still others bid to overcome the painful solitude of death through fusion with a loved one, an ideal, a community, or a God. Regrettably the same practices have secondary damaging aspects. For instance, reliance on religious faith has contributed to individuals being shamed about their body and sexuality inasmuch as they are perceived as indecent or bad and a source of pain, guilt, and embarrassment. In addition, people neglect their lives or misuse their time and energy by presuming that they will live indefinitely. Others commit themselves in loyalty to causes, authorities, or other individuals who stand for ultimate rescuers, renouncing their own identity and autonomy. Others threaten those who maintain dissimilar beliefs, causing discrimination, ethnic cleansing, and even warfare.

Coming to terms with the reality of death turns out to be the only sustainable option against a life of wishful thinking that ends up in detachment from oneself and others. As we get familiar with handling death anxiety, we appreciate life more, feel confident, become open to attachment, and resolve to live in the most pleasant way possible.

References

"On the Nature of Things": Translated by Ronald Latham.

"such as inner conflicts": 1. Greenberg, J, Koole, S L, & Pyszczynski, T (2004). *Handbook of experimental existential psychology.* New York: Guilford. 2. Tomer A (Ed.), *Death attitudes and the older adult: Theories, concepts, and applications.* New York, US: Brunner-Routledge. 3. Weems, C F, Costa, et al. (2004). *Existential Anxiety Questionnaire (EAQ) Development and Scoring Information.* 4. Weems, C F, Costa, N M, Dehon, C, & Berman, S L (2004). *Tillich's Paul. Theory of existential anxiety: A preliminary conceptual and empirical analysis.*

"disable the effectiveness of them": Maxfield, Molly & Greenberg, et al. (2014). *Increases in Generative Concern among Older Adults Following Reminders of Mortality.* International journal of aging & human development.

"Converging evidence supports": Schimel, Jeff, Hayes, et al., *Worldview Threat Increases Death-Thought Accessibility (2007).* Article in Journal of Personality and Social Psychology, June 2007. *Threatening ealth messages:* Robertson J, Jay J, and Welch S (1997). *Can data collection during the grieving process be justifiable?*

"To have feelings of self-worth": 1. Sedikides, C, Gregg, et al. (2007). *The importance of being.* 2. Taylor, S E, Lerner, J S, et al. 2003a, 2003b). *Affirming a positive view.* 3. Sherman, D A K, Nelson, L D, & Steele, C M (2000). *Do messages about health risks threaten the self?*

"espoused by their culture": Jamie Arndt and Matthew Vess (2008*). Tales from Existential Oceans: Terror Management Theory and How the Awareness of Our Mortality Affects Us All.* University of Missouri, Columbia.

"People may be disposed of": 1. Arndt, J, Allen, J J B & Greenberg, J (2001). *Traces of terror: Subliminal death primes and facial electromyographic indices of affect. Motivation and Emotion, 25.* 2. Arndt, J, & Greenberg, J (1999). *The effects of a self-esteem boost and mortality salience on responses to boost relevant and irrelevant worldview threats.* Personality and Social Psychology Bulletin, 25. 3. Arndt, J, Greenberg, J, et al. (2002). *To belong or not to belong, that is the question: Terror management and identification with gender and ethnicity.* Journal of Personality and Social Psychology, 83.

"some kind of resolution": Becker, Ernest (1973). *The Denial of Death.*

"The current findings back up": Clay D Routledge, Jamie Arndt (2009). *Creative Terror Management: Creativity as a Facilitator of Cultural Exploration after Mortality Salience.* PSPB, Vol. 35 No. 4, April 2009.

"could throw off the load": Lucretius, *On the Nature of Things.* Translated by Ronald Latham.

"they are worthy members": 1. Belk, R W (1985). *Materialism: Trait Aspects of Living in the Material World.* Journal of Consumer Research, 14. 2. Carver, Charles S and Baird, Eryn (1995). *The American Dream Revisited: Is It What You Want or Why You Want It That Matters?* 3. Kasser, Tim and Ryan Richard M (1996). *Further Examining the American Dream: Differential Correlates of Intrinsic and Extrinsic Goals.* First Published March 1, Research Article. 4. Schmuck, Peter and Kasser, Tim and Ryan, Richard M (1999). *Intrinsic and Extrinsic*

Goals: Their Structure and Relationship to Well-Being in German and U.S. College Students. 5. Richins, M L and Dawson, S (1992). *A Consumer Values Orientation for Materialism and Its Measurement: Scale Development and Validation.* Journal of Consumer Research, 19.

"the emphasis on wealth": 1. Helga Dittmar, Rod Bond, Megan Hurst, Tim Kasser (2014). *The Relationship between Materialism and Personal Well-Being: A Meta-Analysis.* Article (PDF Available) in Journal of Personality and Social Psychology 107(5):879-924. 2. Haris Dimitriadis (2017). *Epicurus and the Pleasant Life: A Philosophy of Nature.* 1st Edition.

"children are only capable of": 1. Robert W Firestone, Ph.D. (2018). *Death Anxiety.* Psychology Today 2. Solomon, S, Greenberg, J, & Pyszczynski, T A (2015). *The worm at the core: On the role of death in life.* New York: Random House.

"The mortality salience hypothesis": Jamie Arndt and Matthew Vess (2008). *Tales from Existential Oceans: Terror Management Theory and How the Awareness of Our Mortality Affects Us All.* University of Missouri, Columbia.

"we must disapprove and fight": 1. Florian V, Mikulincer M, and Hirschberger G (2002). *The anxiety-buffering function of close relationships: evidence that relationship commitment acts as a terror management mechanism.* Jour. Pers. Soc. Psychol. Apr; 82. 2. Greenberg, Jeff L and Pyszczynski, et al. (1990). *Evidence for Terror Management Theory II: The Effects of Mortality Salience on Reactions to Those Who Threaten or Bolster the Cultural Worldview.* 3. Elliott, Robert K and Greenberg, L S and Lietaer, G (2004). *Research on experiential psychotherapies.* In: Bergin and Garfield's Handbook of Psychotherapy and Behavior Chang 9e. John Wiley & Sons Inc., New York, USA. 4. Cohen F, Solomon S, Maxfield M, Pyszczynski T, Greenberg J (2004). *Fatal*

attraction: the effects of mortality salience on evaluations of charismatic, task-oriented, and relationship-oriented leaders. Psychol. Sci. Dec.; 15(12). 5. Mikulincer, Mario and Shaver, Philip R (2012). *An attachment perspective on psychopathology.* World Psychiatry. Feb; 11(1). 6. Becker, Ernest (1973). *The Denial of Death.*

"the cultural hero-system": Becker, Ernest (1973). *The Denial of Death.*

"Even believing in a God": Elisabeth Kübler-Ross (2008). *On Death and Dying.*

"religious mortality comfort has been diminishing": 1. Jong, Jonathan, Halberstadt, Jamin (2016). *Death Anxiety and Religious Belief: An Existential Psychology of Religion.* 2. Elisabeth Kübler-Ross (2008). *On Death and Dying.*

"the fatality of death": 1. Greenberg, J, & Koole, S L, & Pyszczynski, T (2004). *Handbook of experimental existential psychology.* New York: Guilford. 2. Tomer, A, Eliason, G T, & Wong, P T P (2008). *Existential and spiritual issues in death attitudes.* New York, NY. 3. Weems, C F, & Costa, N M, & Dehon, C, & Berman, S L (2004). *Existential Anxiety Question-naire (EAQ) Development and Scoring Information from Paul Tillich's theory of existential anxiety: A preliminary conceptual and empirical analysis.* Anxiety, Stress, & Coping, 17. 4. Solomon, S, Greenberg, J, & Pyszczynski, T (1991). *A Terror Management Theory of Social Behavior: The Psychological Functions of Self-Esteem and Cultural Worldviews.* 5. Solomon, Sheldon & Greenberg, Jeff (2015). *The Worm at the Core: On the Role of Death in Life*

"studies show that patients": Furer, P, Walker, J R, Chartier, M J, & Stein, M. B. (1997). *Hypochondriacal concerns and somatization in panic disorder.*

"fear of dying from a heart attack": 1. Fleet, Richard & Beitman, Bernard D (1998*). Cardiovascular death from panic disorder and panic-like anxiety: A critical review of the literature.* Article Literature Review in Journal of Psychosomatic Research 44(1). 2. Clare L and Jones R S (2008). *Errorless learning in the rehabilitation of memory impairment: a critical review.* Neuropsychol. Rev. 2008 Mar; 18(1).

"separation anxiety disorder and agoraphobia": 1. Vaccaro, L, Jones, M, Menzies, R, & St Clare, T (2010). *Danger Ideation Reduction Therapy (DIRT) for obsessive–compulsive checkers: A comprehensive guide to treatment.* Bowen Hills: Australian Academic Press. 2. Baldwin D S, & Gordon R, & Abelli M, & Pini S (2016). *The separation of adult separation anxiety disorder.* CNS Spectr. 2016 Aug; 21(4)

"opposition to others": Becker, Ernest (1985). *Escape from Evil.*

"Obsessive thoughts and practice": 1. Vaccaro, L, Jones, M, Menzies, R, & St Clare, T (2010). *Danger Ideation Reduction Therapy (DIRT) for obsessive–compulsive checkers: A comprehensive guide to treatment.* Bowen Hills: Australian Academic Press. 2. Strachan, E, Schimel, J, et al. (2007). *Terror mismanagement: Evidence that mortality salience exacerbates phobic and compulsive behaviors.* Personality and Social Psychology Bulletin, 33, 1137–1151.

"research has shown": 1. Robert W Firestone, Ph.D. (2018). *Death Anxiety. Psychology Today* 2. Florian, V., & Mikulincer, M. (2004). *A multifaceted perspective on the existential meanings, manifestations, and consequences of the fear of personal death.* In J Greenberg, S L Koole, & T Pyszczynski (Eds.), Handbook of experimental existential psychology (pp. 54–70). New York: Guilford. 3. Hart, J, & Goldenberg, J L (2008). *A terror management perspective on spirituality and the problem of the body.* In

A Tomer, G T Eliason, & P T P Wong (Eds.), Existential and spiritual issues in death attitudes (pp. 91–113). New York: Lawrence Erlbaum. 4. Kastenbaum, R (2000). *The psychology of death* (3rd ed.). New York: Springer. 5. Solomon, S, Greenberg, J, & Pyszczynski, T A (2015). *The worm at the core: On the role of death in life*. New York: Random House.

CHAPTER 5

PESSIMISM

"The wise man neither seeks to escape life nor fears the cessation of life, for neither does life offend him nor does the absence of life seem to be any evil."

—Epicurus, *Letter to Menoeceus*

Epicurus was in opposition to *the pessimist philosophers of his time*. Despite starting off from similar positions to those of Epicurus—namely that pleasure is the only good—the pessimists concluded that pleasure rarely reaches its fullness. They argued that more often than not, the desire for it leads to frustration, while its enjoyment ends up in saturation and disgust; in life, pain is greater than pleasure, and happiness is never realized: happiness is a fallacy. Pursuing happiness, or just pleasure, is something hollow and contradictory since in reality we will always find more pain than pleasure and there is only one way to feel less pain: to be indifferent to pleasure and to the sources of it, to diminish our sensitivity to it, and nullify the desire of it. Indifference of, and renunciation to pleasure, are the only means of securing comfort in life. Worst of all, these same pessimists claimed that life is no more attractive than death and those who are tired of pursuing pleasure can be healed through death; pleasure, which is considered the ultimate positive purpose of life, is inaccessible, and the least we should do is to live in a kind of ascetic denial. In short, life is worthy of death and death is worthy of life.

47

Modern pessimists move along the same lines. They argue that life is futile. Both personally and broadly speaking, life is meaningless essentially because of the fact of suffering. It would be better if there was nothing. We came from nothing after aeons of time and before long we will return to nothing. Each moment of life is transitory and fleeting and hastily becomes the past; in other words, it disappears into blankness. The clock of our lives is slowly counting down. In reaction, we might naturally do our best to enjoy the present, but since the present so swiftly grows into the past, it is not deserving of any significant effort. Such a life is one of struggling all the time for what can rarely be achieved or what, when achieved, upsets without delay. Thinking about the role it plays in our lives, we discover that we did not in fact enjoy it, but rather faced it as simply the way to the future, and yet all our struggling is futile since we inevitably die. Suffering and adversity are the common pattern in life, not the deviation. We can notice this by bearing in mind that happiness or pleasure invariably entail some unhappiness or pain being brought to an end; and furthermore, pleasure is not usually as pleasant as we anticipated, while pain is usually much worse than conceived. Yet we are unable to cease time; we slowly but surely realize many of our hopes will never be fulfilled, and we acknowledge that day by day we grow older and weaker, resulting in an inescapable fate. If we reflect on the course of our lives from birth to death, we become aware of the vanity of life. Suffering, the transience of the present, the understanding of death—and the fact of death itself—all diminish the hope of a meaningful life. In other words, the purpose of our being is non-being and therefore it may have been better if we had never lived at all.

Pessimists tend to focus on the negatives in life in general and anticipate undesirable outcomes in most circumstances. The main causes of pessimism are tracked down to bad past experiences, a defeatist belief system, fatalistic religious faith, low self-esteem, health-related problems, and coping with pessimistic people. If we want to deal with pessimism there is nothing better we can do other than fixing our belief system, building self-esteem, and spending more time with optimists.

A pessimistic or optimistic attitude to life greatly affects a person's fear of death. The awareness of the inevitability of death leads individuals with a negative attitude to live their life in an existential crisis with an intense fear of death. In contrast, optimists think in a positive manner, look upon things in an affirmative way, build up self-confidence, find meaning in life, and ameliorate death anxiety.

Epicurus appreciated *positive thinking* and a positive attitude in the pursuit of happiness by stressing that the steady state of wellness and the certain hope that it will last longer offers more confident joy to those who know how to assess things correctly. All contemporary studies confirm this assumption. It turns out that an optimistic attitude transmits a message to the brain that the future will be secure and therefore it can confidently channel energy resources in search of pleasure, creativity, and development. On the contrary, as long as pessimistic thoughts predominate, the mind is in a defensive mode, wasting energy resources by enhancing muscle power to defend the self against imagined or actual risks. In such conditions the mind creates strong neural circuits to support the idea of the vanity of life and consequently of the futility of pursuing any goals. Similar are the consequences when we question our abilities and conclude that we cannot do anything well or that everything will go wrong.

Negative thoughts are doubtless the most salient sources of human misery by inflicting long-term stress; they set the mind in a mode of prolonged red alert, deplete the body of valuable energy resources, and gradually lead to exhaustion and collapse. A painful consequence of this development is the acute disruption of the emotional functions leading to panic, anxiety, and depression. To confront the phenomenon of negative thoughts we have to reconsider our habits and beliefs and train ourselves to think positively. The Epicurean tenets are a valuable source of optimistic beliefs for those committed to transforming themselves.

References

"the pessimist philosophers of his time": Hegesias of Cyrene. Wikipedia

"Modern pessimists": 1. Arthur Schopenhauer (2004). *The Essays of Arthur Schopenhauer: Studies in Pessimism.* Translated by T Bailey Saunders, M A. 2. Albert Camus (1955). *The Myth of Sisyphus.*

"positive thinking": 1. Seligman, Martin (2011). *Authentic Happiness.* 2. Seligman, Martin (2018). *Learned Optimism.* 3. Csikszentmihalyi, Mihaly (1998). *Finding Flow: The Psychology of Engagement with Everyday Life.* 4. Csikszentmihalyi, Mihaly (2009). *Flow: The Psychology of Optimal Experience.* 5. Csikszentmihalyi, Mihaly and Hunter, Jeremy (2003). Happiness in Everyday Life.*

"Negative thoughts": 1. LeDoux, J E (1996). *The Emotional Brain.* New York: Simon and Schuster Paperbacks. 2. LeDoux, J E (1998). *Fear and the brain: Where have we been, and where are we going? Biol. Psychiatr.* 1998; 44:1229–38. [PubMed].

CHAPTER 6

THERAPY FOR THE FEAR OF DEATH

"So death, the most terrifying of ills, is nothing to us, since so long as we exist, death is not with us; but when death comes, then we do not exist. It does not then concern either the living or the dead, since for the former it is not, and the latter are no more."

—Epicurus, *Letter to Menoeceus*

Philosophy cures human maladies, maladies generated by deluded convictions. Its reasoning is to the soul as the physician's medication is to the body. It can cure, and it is to be assessed by its competence to cure. The hardest problem for it to tackle is treating death anxiety. The Epicurean philosophy claims that it is the most suitable therapy for a fear of death. It recommends that we should come face to face with death in the same manner that we face any fear. We should consent to our end of life and habituate ourselves with the reality of it. Acknowledging and adopting the certainty of death can bring a sense of appreciation to life and its pleasures. It could also take away superfluous distress by the realization that it is not death that is important, but how we deal with it in life. While death annihilates us, our view of it may come to our rescue.

Efforts to flee death anxiety often result in emotional conflict and become apparent as self-defeating reactions, dependency behaviors, or at variance with these, and may include participation in dangerous hobbies or actions of heroism and defiance, *sexual hyperactivity, and unfaithfulness.* When we defy the fear of death, we are more competent to stand up to death with tranquility, live in the here and now, and encounter the pleasure and suffering of being without having recourse to daydreaming and self-deception. By becoming more free and helpless, we are in a position to value the joys of life.

Several contemporary therapies have been developed to treat death anxiety, among them, the existential-humanistic and *cognitive-behavior therapy* approaches are the most commonly applied. The existential-humanistic treatment acknowledges that individuals facing death experience physical pain as well as psychological distress and existential suffering. As such, treatment is focused on *bolstering meaning* and spiritual well-being, increasing psychosocial support, building and maintaining relationships, improving coping skills, resolving unconscious and conscious conflicts, providing education about depressive symptoms and possible triggers, and changing dysfunctional behavior patterns. Similarly, *evidence confirms the potential* of existential approaches to support other treatments, such as cognitive-behavior therapy. Although cognitive and existential therapies have largely been regarded as diverse and incompatible, integration of these two approaches has been found to refine the treatment of death anxiety and psychopathology (the scientific study of mental disorders), with a focus on improving self-esteem and meaning. In addition, the so-called *acceptance and commitment therapy* includes tasks that explicitly confront death, such as writing your own eulogy and choosing the words for your tombstone.

The Epicurean therapy of fear of death consisted of a four-step course of action: disclosure of the exact cause of the fear through comprehensive discussion and exposure; acquaintance with philosophical therapeutic arguments; intellectual exercises such as concentration, meditations and remembrances of pleasant things; and lastly, developing friendship. The first and last steps involve self-motivation and human interaction and therefore we will only deal with the cognitive part of the therapy in this book.

Arguments to tame the fear of death

The fear of death is external to human nature

It is inflicted on us by painful experiences and erroneous societal influences. It is then within the scope of the philosophy to heal this agitation of the soul from the terror of death the same way it does with any acquired human fear. Epicurus' understanding of the fear of death coincides with contemporary approaches, suggesting that *in our subconscious* we are immortal. It is indeed impossible to imagine our own death and whenever we attempt to do so we are in fact present as spectators. *We can't imagine how* or what we would be like once we are dead without being able to think or see, for example.

The fear of death is irrational

All of our logical decisions rest on and relate to sensation. Therefore, it is irrational to claim that death is evil for us since we will never sense it; on the contrary, it will be a deprivation of sensation, and for that reason it is of no concern to us. On top of that, inasmuch as death is not hurting when present, it is not reasonable to be afraid of it when it is expected. Thus, if nothing can be good or bad for as long as we do not sense it, how can death be of any concern to us? The wise human being neither rejects life nor fears death.

Death is the final atomic dissolution of man

In physics the entire world is constructed of atoms and empty space. As mentioned earlier, according to neuroscience, the soul is the emotional circuitry of the brain, responsible for the generation and memorization of emotions. It is of organic nature and consequently has an atomic structure. Epicurus shared similar views but placed the soul-emotional center in the chest rather than the brain. Nonetheless, he is right on the core premise that the soul cannot be made of empty space but of atoms since it interacts very closely with the body. He is also right by claiming that these atomic structures are fragile, and at the time of our death they cease to function and consequently the soul loses all the powers it had while living. This implies that we will be unable to feel any emotional or physical pain and therefore it is foolish to be preoccupied with the notion of death while alive.

The symmetry argument

The Epicurean philosopher-poet asserts that *when we shall be no more*, when the union of body and spirit has been disrupted, no hazard will happen to us anymore. If we look back at the eternity that passed before we were born, we will realize that our own life had been nothing in relation to the preexisted life. *This resembles a mirror* that Nature holds up to *us*, which reflects the time that shall be after we are dead. Surprisingly though, there seems to be an asymmetry in our attitude towards our prenatal nonexistence and our posthumous nonexistence. While in each of these periods of time we do not exist, we fear our later limit of life—that is, death—but share no similar feeling towards our earlier limit of life—i.e. birth. Rather, given the symmetry between the two temporal limits of our existence, our attitudes towards our birth and death should also be symmetrical, and since there is nothing frightening in the earlier temporal limit of our existence, we should also not fear the later temporal limit of it. Both sides of life are equally blocked to our fears and desires and consequently we must turn away our gaze from the infinity of time that lies beyond the end of our life, the same way we do with the infinity of time that preexisted our birth.

Death in no way deprives anything from the dead

There are also those who embrace the modern cultural idea of deprivation, claiming that death harms the deceased by depriving him of possible future goods. The classic deprivation notion of the good life is described as an existentialist-like perspective in which human life is an endless work-in-progress—in a sense, one is consistently an observer of the story of his or her life as it develops on the way to the future. Bundled up with this view is a high appreciation for human desire; death, on such a consideration, is seen as a lost chance, or as no more chances left, and as the collapse of one's life's work. The deprivation argument also highlights the question of premature death by stressing the importance of age. Premature death, people claim, is worse than a late death; the number of good life years lost matter to the 'badness' of death. The death of infants or victims of war and accidents, for example, is worse than the death of those dying due to old age. To all such claims, Epicurus responds that the special features of death are of no concern to the dead; what matters is the mere fact of death and nothing more. Certainly, before anything else, deprivation advocates have to explain how, when, and to whom the harm occurs. Most probably they unconsciously reflect their own thoughts and feelings to the deceased or else they assume that something living remains after death. In such a case, they are in the grip of an inconsistent mental picture of the event. Although they actually believe that the person ends at death, they also imagine a surviving subject who is pained and grieved by damage to his corpse and by the loss to himself of the good things in life, such as children, home, various pleasures and activities. By imagining the dead grieving, they mistakenly endow him with life.

Besides, *it is not the fulfillment of hopes* either that confers meaning on life, but rather the way in which we live at any given moment. In other words, the completeness of our life lies in our state of being, not in the completion of projects, fulfillment of desires, and hopes. The good life is not a process on the way to some further goal beyond itself, susceptible to disruption before it can reach that goal. If it is there it is there, and nothing beyond that but that itself is the end. By encouraging us to reconsider our values and commit ourselves to self-sufficient pleasures, Epicurus aims to shield our lives from the accidents of life.

Reconsidering our philosophy of life

The philosophy of Epicurus goes far beyond a hedonistic attitude to life. In essence, it introduces a therapy for treating anxiety that brings about peace of mind. In order to free mankind from all that inflicts distress on the soul, Epicurus affirms that gods are fearless because they neither manage the universe or bother about people. With regard to death, he claims that the soul does not survive the body and that death is not a happening within life. With regard to desires, he suggests rejecting those that are neither natural nor necessary, such as wealth, fame and power, and satisfy with prudence those of our desires that are natural but not necessary, such as amusement and luxuries. Above all, we are to satisfy those desires that are vital for the continuation of our life, such as food, water, and shelter.

Humans, like all other living beings, are always attracted by pleasure. If we are after wisdom, this is simply because it increases pleasure and contributes to peace of mind. All in all, Epicurus suggests that to liberate our souls from distress, we need to totally restructure our lives, especially with regard to our attitude toward time and pleasure. Indeed, much of mankind is obsessed with unbounded needless desires to acquire wealth, fame, and power. What is common to all these desires is that they are impossible to be fulfilled in the present by the average individual and whenever they are, they hardly bring more happiness. This is why, for the Epicureans, mindless people live in hope for the future, and as this is uncertain, they are overwhelmed by fear and worry about the realization of their desires. Therefore, wisdom proposes to put an emphasis on the enjoyment of the pleasure of the present. However, to be able to do so we have to revise our understanding of pleasure and time in order to incorporate in them the Epicurean maxim that the quality of pleasure depends neither on the number of desires it satisfies, nor on the duration of them. It can be secured simply by the enjoyment of natural and necessary desires; that is, those desires that are indispensable for the sustenance of life. Such desires can easily be gratified without our having to count on the future for their provision, and without putting too much effort to acquire them. In short, the secret of Epicurean joy and serenity is the experience of infinite pleasure provided by the consciousness of existence, even if it be only for a moment. In the words of an Epicurean saying, the cry of the flesh is not to be hungry, not to be thirsty, not to be cold. Whoever has these things, and hopes to keep on having them, can rival in happiness with Zeus himself. The lack of hunger and thirst is thus the condition for being able to continue to exist and enjoying the awareness of existing.

The Epicureans thought of pleasure as a reality in and for itself, not situated within the confines of time. Indeed, time is not an intrinsic feature of mankind but an acquired capacity of consciousness. As proof, let's get back to animals and little children to figure out how unaware they are of time and how long it takes for children to get a grasp on its passage and their growing up. Are we not allowed to assume that our emotions, such as our inherent faculty of feeling pleasure and pain, are also timeless for so long as we are immersed in them? In the midst of the flow of pleasure, we are cut off from thoughts and perception of time for as long as we are totally absorbed in what we are doing, and therefore one single instant of happiness is enough to give such pleasure as infinity does.

This sensation is reinforced by the amazing quality of feelings to have limits. Once thirsty, we need so much water that no pain from thirst is present. By drinking more, we add nothing to the pleasure of satisfying our thirst. Moreover, the pleasure of a meal is not enhanced by prolonging it but rather by emphasizing on the quality of the food and the conditions surrounding it. Again, the pleasure of an artistic performance reaches an apex beyond which any prolongation of the performance decreases rather than increases its value. These examples show that pleasure has an upper limit and once that is reached, no additional action can affect it anymore. In other words, happiness is an entirely internal mental process that gets its maximum expression by organic functions. Once happy, we need no more of pleasure. This conclusion contradicts common sense that suggests it is logic, rather than feelings, that has limits. To see the falsehood of this assertion let's consider how wrong our logical valuations might be and how limitless our search for riches, power, and fame could be. Spirit has no limits. It could easily extend from nothingness to infinity. On the contrary, feelings do have internal boundaries. Once we enjoy peace of mind we have attained the climax of pleasure and there is no better state to reach than that.

The immense value in each moment

The view that the world is the outcome of an accident, leaving out all providential mediation, makes for undiluted pleasure and peace of mind, unchains us from the senseless fear of gods, and encourages people to greet each moment with immense gratitude. It is precisely because our existence is the result of pure chance that *the present moment lasts forever*. In Epicurus, the present moment takes on an infinite value: it contains within it the entire cosmos and all the value and wealth of being. In other words, enjoying the present without thinking about the past or the future does not mean living in total instantaneousness; when we focus our attention on the present, we find out that the present instant is overloaded with meaning by being a transition and a transformation of reality. Such a moment represents a whole past and a whole future. Imagine how a talented painter can capture in an instant the complete view of his subject, enabling the viewer to see both the earlier and the later state of it. The scene may be hooked on for a moment, but that single moment is capable of revealing simultaneously the past, the present, and the future of it. In the same way, the wise man recognizes that each instant of his life is overflowing with meaning; it comprises both the past and the future, not only of him, but also of the universe in which he is immersed.

Pleasure is total and complete at each moment of its duration

To Epicurus, pleasure is timeless. Pleasure is complete at each instance of its time span, and its extension does not alter its fundamental qualities. When pleasure rises to the level that assures peace of mind, *happiness reaches its optimum level,* the so-called ataraxia or state of serenity that cannot be improved on by an extension of its lifetime. In pleasure there is a sort of internal fullness. Genuine pleasure brings *infinity within itself.* On the contrary, the life of an unwise man is fearsome and miserable; it is carried away into the future because the course of his life is dependent on certain future conditions being met. Prudence recommends a major adjustment of attitude toward time by acquiring the skill of enjoying the pleasure of the moment. If the past is hurting, we are to keep away from reflecting on it, as we should also do about the future to the extent it looks unpleasant and hopeless. For what possible reason should I obstruct myself from savoring the present moment as though I am sure of the one that follows, and then waste that one as well in concerns and pointless worries? If the sun shines on me today, why should I become desperate about what happened yesterday? How could I possibly envision the fate of the oncoming day?

The good life is measured not by duration, but by quality

The good life is assessed not by its duration but by its fullness. This attitude presumes a specific capture of pleasure, endorsing that the quality of that pleasure hinges on neither the number of desires it fulfills or on the extent of time it lasts. The finest and most exceptional pleasure then is that which is accompanied to the least extent by worry, and which is very likely to establish peace of mind. Accordingly, the wise man rises above his mortality and he will care not for the long-lasting life but rather the most pleasant one.

Wider viewpoint

Nature's voice asks us to perceive our life from a broader standpoint: when we contemplate our life as one within the whole, two things become apparent. First of all, our personal worries look minuscule; we come to wonder, why should we consume our lives in expectation of our death when there is so much in the world to reflect on? Others have died; birth and death are both global and inevitable; ours is not a particular case. Our worldview opens up. Secondly, when we imagine our death from the perspective of the universe, we conceive that as a necessary development for the conservation of health and life of our planet and the people who live on it. *There is a requirement of matter,* so that ensuing generations may be nurtured. They too, having lived out their lives, will come after us. Generations have arrived, given birth to new ones, and then vanished. For that reason, one thing will never stop emerging from another. Life is no one's exclusive possession. Put briefly, Nature states: this life to which you so obstinately cling is not only a tiny portion of the whole, it is indeed demanded back from you if the whole is to survive. If people never died, that would bring all of Nature to a standstill: no space for childbirth and no reserves for the newly born. Adhering to life by any means is selfishness and misanthropy. With regard to death, there is one inescapable drawback for man: all men must die; there is no escape.

The various stages of life alternate in harmony with each other

Youth replaces childhood, maturity succeeds youth, aging comes after maturity, and aging concludes in death. We are unable to bring back the life that comes to its full end: it is better to die with grace in order to die peacefully. Humans must relay the torch of life from hand to hand to shine its splendor all over the world. Blood must not draw to a close but be eternally circulated in the veins of Mother Nature. The wise man, unable to do otherwise, will endure death the same way he does with all natural hardships: he will face his death with the tranquility of what is inevitable. The more courageous and strong he is, the less we will fear the suffering of dying.

Paying our debt to Nature

The wise man has feelings of astonishment and gratitude to Nature for her function as the creative force in the universe. He does not complain about death or laments with tears for his upcoming demise more than is right because he has enjoyed all the necessary pleasure in life, since there is no more pleasure that Nature can discover for him: all things are forever the same. As a result, Nature is justified to reply in a sharp tone of voice to *those aging who raise their voice* and rally against her, that because they ever wished for what is not present—and despised what is—life has slipped from their grasp unfinished and unsatisfying, and death has taken his stand at their pillow. However, now is time to waive all things unsuited to their age; go, they must—courageous and serene.

The debt to Nature is not to be found merely in nurturing living beings by making life's necessities easy to acquire and those things that are difficult to find unnecessary, but also in her *function as a teacher*. It is Nature that reveals the truth and bestows upon man the means of contact between his soul and the material world. Nature reveals also the true end of living. True justice is again the justice of Nature. The true attitude towards desires consists in recognizing the limits of Nature. The true attitude toward riches and poverty demands knowledge of the wealth of Nature. She is the moral teacher: Nature teaches us to think the gifts of fortune as being of minor value. Nature urges us to realize that life is like a banquet: it has a structure in time that reaches a natural and appropriate termination; its value cannot be prolonged far beyond that without spoiling the value that preceded it. Men should therefore not strive to prolong their lives indefinitely, since this will just spoil the pleasure of the life that they have. As the Epicurean philosopher-poet pronounces, Nature is so eager for men to know the truths of life that she barks it aloud, like a faithful dog that is eager to give warning.

Man is endowed with this very act of annihilation

Our life is indeed full of acts of minor deaths. Fainting or being under an anesthetic during surgery are examples of minor deaths. Dreamless sleep is equally a microscopic death. Although one may argue that sleep is a pleasure in and of itself, this is not so, because the so-called pleasure of sleep is not felt during sleep, but after waking up. Deep dreamless sleep involves total loss of consciousness and sensation, and what has no memories, thoughts, and feelings is similar to being dead.

Death is ever present in life. It really has nothing terrible in it. For the intellect, it is reasonable and almost useful, for the feeling is akin to nothing.

Any desire not confirmed by Nature itself must be rejected

The desire for immortality, for example, is one that should be discarded in pursuit of living a better, more pleasurable life. The Epicurean philosopher-poet declares that the wise man is neither jealous of the supposed happiness of immortality, nor of the wreaths awarded to poets, nor the statues erected in honor of the conquerors. He does not rely upon future events but looks forward to them in peace. We must remember that Epicurus says the future is neither entirely ours, nor is it not, so that we should not expect with full confidence that it will come or be desperate that it will never come.

Death is bad for others but not for the deceased

Frequently, the perspective that our loved ones weep at our death intensifies the idea that our dying hurts us rather than them. Similarly, our sorrow at imagining our loved ones suffering due to our absence is not a reliable alibi to believe our death is harmful to us: the disappointment our death inflicts on them by no means has an effect on us, and our anticipated anguish is senseless. What's more, their sadness will be moderated by the reality that our death is not harmful to us.

Pain is the evil

When we say we are afraid of death, we are deceiving ourselves. In reality it is not death that we are afraid of, but it is the pain of the process of dying that we find frightening. We simply lack the bravery to face an approaching death, a virtue that neither the Epicurean philosophy or indeed any other philosophy can offer. Undoubtedly death is not a good thing, but we know that it is not bad either, and we recognize on the other hand that occasionally life may turn out sore: it is then obvious that between the misery of pain and the nothingness of death, nothingness is preferable. That is why we sometimes endure some pain in anticipation of more pleasure: pain, although ugly in itself, is then transformed into something good. Even more than that, death—which is not bad in itself—can be good in so far as it takes away more pain than pleasure.

The pain that often precedes death is a fact that the wise man acknowledges without reservations and suggests that people should tolerate this last pain with the same courage he does for any pain. As soon as he puts up with this pain, a new period will open up for him: the complete anesthesia, the annihilation, which no longer causes fear either to the courageous man or to the coward or to any human being. From the point of view of feeling, death is neither pleasant nor unpleasant, because it is the elimination of feelings; in addition, it is the rational point of view of the intellect because it is concomitant to the logic of Nature. Being is a state that we must accept as it is in its relative perfection. It is a master-piece, a poem that we do not embellish by dragging it out.

The wise man is conscious that each new day that dawns may be the last for him and salutes each additional moment as if it were an incredible stroke of luck. He enjoys the uniqueness of life and the fullness of the present instant. He is well acquainted with the reality that we are only born once, twice is not allowed, and that we shall be no more for all eternity. He eludes the sting of fear of death by familiarizing himself with the notion that 'death is nothing to us'. He departs life as a spectator and leaves the theater having enjoyed the pleasure of the performance.

Techniques to overcome the fear of death

The arguments employed in fighting the fear of death were an essential part of the curriculum of studies of the Epicurean school. The theoretical education was complemented by practices aiming at self-knowledge, removal of the corrupt beliefs, and assimilation of the healthy tenets of the school. Some of the techniques taught included learning what to read, developing the capacity of dialogue, practicing meditation, turning the mind away from unpleasant thoughts, embracing our own mortality, learning not to fear death, having the capacity to develop friendship, developing the courage to expose the troubling aspects of the psyche, such as worries, fears, and insecurities, and so on.

Learning what to read

To gain knowledge is not an end in itself but a channel of understanding ourselves and ridding us of the inessential to discover what is essential beneath. Even the written master-pieces of philosophy are not important in themselves but should be valued in the extent that they contribute to wellbeing. One reads and writes philosophy not so that one can be clever about it, but because the practice of reading and writing itself is directed towards teaching and learning the way to cast out the *suffering of the soul* and enjoy pleasure. Theory has to be clearly and decidedly put in the service of obtaining the serenity of the soul.

Developing the capacity of dialogue

Spiritual enterprise is never a lonely affair. For this reason, the ancient philosophical schools were often communal. Only he who is capable of a genuine touch with another is capable of an authentic encounter with himself, and the converse is equally true. By questioning and investigating each other, carefully anatomizing and examining ideas, detecting inconsistencies, never abusing but always inquiring for what we may consent on, we can slowly obtain deeper conception and insight into ourselves and others. The procedure calls for heeding with empathy, searching new ideas and outlooks, delivering new understandings, and reinforcing relationships within the community.

Meditation of Epicurean precepts

Spiritual exercises are required for the healing of the soul. The Epicureans advise us to meditate upon and assimilate, day and night, brief aphorisms or summaries that will allow us to keep the fundamental dogmas at hand.

Some of these dogmas are suitable in learning to concentrate on the miniscule while others can assist with practicing mental flight in the cosmos. In particular, the transformation of our view of the world is intimately linked to exercises that involve concentrating on the miniscule moment. Such exercises are intended to turn ourselves away from the future and past in order to define the moment. Concentration on the minuscule moment is always bearable and controllable; it releases the mind from the burden and prejudices of the past, as well as the worries about the future, in order to acquire inner freedom and peace. Along with the concentration on the miniscule instant, Epicurean physics enables the mind to open up to the infinity of time and space. Our mind can plunge its gaze far beyond the boundaries of our planet to contemplate the infinity of space-time in its bright, eternal tranquility, unconcerned by mundane affairs. Our thoughts can get in touch with the cosmic sentiment, become mindful of the infinite value of each instant, and welcome each moment of our being within the perspective of the cosmos.

More on meditations follows in the next chapter.

Remembrance of good things

Memory performs a diverse role as a spiritual exercise. In the first place there is the memorization of the doctrines and sayings of the philosophy; and there is also the memory of beloved friends and fellow philosophers. When we hold on to the memory of our lost friends, they reside within us and are capable of uplifting our spirits more so than when they breathed and walked the Earth. The exercise of turning the mind away from displeasing thoughts towards pleasant ones is very helpful in coping with the fear of death. It can equally become an integral part of our daily practices, enhancing our valuation of the natural good of pleasure and dissuading the natural evil of pain.

Learning not to fear death

When we get used to the idea of death, we are either able to get over it or come to peace with it, so the phobia of the event no longer controls our life. Circumstances of incurable illness provide an opportunity to contemplate and share thoughts and feelings on death and dying. This is especially true if the dying person is able to work through his own grief and show by example how one can die with equanimity, he will be of great help to his loved ones in their effort to bear their own sorrow with courage and dignity.

Developing friendships

Intimate connections help us cope with the fear of death. We should therefore treasure our relationships with family, nurture old friendships, and develop new ones. Friendship enables people to be open to each other without reservations and be assured that their confessions will stay confidential. Friends don't have to worry about true friends talking behind their back because they will stick up for each other even in their absence.

Learning to expose ourselves

Epicurus was the first philosopher ever to discover the importance of the unconscious functions of the mind who also made use of practices aimed at curing the unconscious pains of the soul. The therapeutic course involved long in-depth discussions with teachers and peers in a friendly environment of trust and affection in order for the disciples to promptly expose themselves. The disciples could *be wrong about their health* in many ways. They could suppose that they were fine when actually they were not. This may owe to the fact that their disease had not yet revealed itself through visible signs and symptoms, or it may be on account of not having felt any better before. The sage is well aware that usually the trouble lies in the cognitive makeup of the person, especially in his beliefs, desires, and preferences. He is also thoughtful about any statement made by the disciple knowing that the very same issues reported are the ones that are—or might be—ailing. And still, how can the sage make them out but by urging a pupil to talk? The sage will have to question him over and over again to single out the healthy parts from the corrupt. Certainly, no piece of the self is immune to reason, but reasoning must search thoroughly in order to get in touch with the troubled parts of the soul. In many respects, the challenge undertaken by the sage resembles the challenge of confronting a psychologist or psychiatrist who tries to deal with the root cause of mental disturbance or disease.

Embracing our own mortality

Coping with the fear of death cannot be done on a mass level by virtue of the fact that societies are tuned into the denial of death. Unfortunately, everyone has to make an effort on his own. Unconsciously, we postpone such questions and topics until we are forced to face them through an illness of our own or the death of a loved one. Yet it would be very helpful for us if we made an all-out effort to deal with our anxieties surrounding our own death and ask ourselves what we as individuals can do about all of this. Embracing our mortality in a genuine way will enable us to grasp what our death means to us and how it affects our lives. Instead of trying to find out the least harmful way to deny our death, it would be better to question ourselves about how we can connect to it in a way that affirms our lives.

References

"sexual hyperactivity, and unfaithfulness": Watter D N (2018). *Existential Issues in Sexual Medicine: The Relation between Death Anxiety and Hypersexuality.* Sex Med Rev. 2018 Jan.

"Cognitive-behavior therapy": 1. Beck, A T, & Weishaar, M E (1995). *Cognitive therapy. In R J Corsini, & D Wedding (Eds.),* Current psychotherapies (pp. 229–261). Itasca, I L: Peacock. 2. Ottens, A J, & Hanna, F J (1998). *Cognitive and existential therapies: Toward an integration.* Psychotherapy: Theory, Research, Practice, Training, 35, 312–324. 3. Safran, J D (1996). *Book review.* Journal of Psychotherapy Integration, 6, 179–181. 4. Waltz, T J, & Hayes, S,C (2010). *Acceptance and commitment therapy. 5.* N Kazantzis, M A Reinecke, et al. *Cognitive and behavioral theories in clinical practice.* New York, NY: Guilford Press.

"bolstering meaning": 1. Chochinov, Harvey Max and Kristjanson, Linda J, and Breitbart, William, et al. (2011). *The effect of dignity therapy on distress and end-of-life experience in terminally ill patients: a randomized controlled trial.* Lancet Oncol. 2011 Aug; 12(8): 753–762. 2. Johns, S A (2013). *Translating Dignity Therapy into practice: Effects and lessons learned.* Omega: Journal of Death and Dying, 67.

"evidence confirms the potential": 1. Breitbart W, Rosenfeld B, et al. (2000). *Depression, hopelessness, and desire for hastened death in terminally ill patients with cancer.* Oncology (Williston Park). 2000 Nov; 14(11). 2. Kash KM, Holland J C, et al. *Stress and burnout in oncology.* Oncology (Williston Park). 2000 Nov; 14(11):1621–33.

"acceptance and commitment therapy": 1. Hayes, J, Schimel, J, & Williams, T J (2008). *Fighting death with death: The buffering effects of learning that worldview violators have died.* Psychological Science, 19, 501–507. 2. Hayes, S C, & Smith, S (2005). *Get out of your mind and into your life: The new Acceptance and Commitment Therapy.* Oakland, CA: New Harbinger Publications, Inc.

"in our subconscious": Freud, S (1952). *Thoughts for the times on war and death.* E C Mayne. Trans. In R Hutchins (Ed.).

"We can't imagine how": Freud, S (1955). *On Transience.* In J Strachey ed. and trans. Standard Edition of the Complete Psychological Works of Sigmund Freud. Vol. 14. London: Hogarth Press, 1955, pp. 304–307. Originally published 1915.

"when we shall be no more": Lucretius. *On the Nature of Things.* Translated by Cyril Bailey (1910) Oxford press, p134 l 3.

"This resembles a mirror": Lucretius. *On the Nature of things.* Translated by Cyril Bailey (1910) Oxford press, p138, l 23.

"There are also those": 1. Nussbaum, M C (1994). *The Therapy of Desire: Theory and Practice in Hellenistic Ethics.* Princeton. 2. Nagel, T (1979). *Death.* In Mortal Questions, 1–10. Cambridge: Cambridge University Press. 3. Pitcher, G (1984). *The Misfortunes of the Dead.* American Philosophical Quarterly 21(2): 183-88. 4. Feinberg, G. (1984). *Harm to Others.* Oxford: Oxford University Press. Reprinted in part in Fischer. 5. Luper-Foy, S (1987). *Annihilation.* Philosophical Quarterly 37(148):233-252. Reprinted in Fischer. 6. Feldman, F (1991). *Some Puzzles about the Harm of Death.* Philosophical Review 100(2):205-27.

"it is not the fulfillment of hopes": Rosenbaum, S. E. (1990). *Epicurus on Pleasure and the Complete Life.* Monist 73:21-45.

"the present moment lasts forever": 1. Horace. *The Epistles of Horace Ode 1.11.* 2. Horace and Radice Betty. *The Complete Odes and Epodes.* 3. Pierre Hadot (1995). *Philosophy as a Way of Life: Spiritual Exercises from Socrates to Foucault.* Translated by Michael Chase.

"happiness reaches its optimum level": Haris Dimitriadis (2017). *Epicurus and the Pleasant Life: A Philosophy of Nature.* 1st Edition.

"infinity within itself": Principal Doctrine 20.

"There is a requirement of matter": Lucretius, *On the Nature of Things.*

"those aging who raise their voice": Lucretius, *On the Nature of Things.*

"function as a teacher": Norman Wentworth Dewitt (1954). Epicurus and His Philosophy, University of Minnesota Press, Minneapoli.

"suffering of the soul": Martha C Nussbaum (1994). *The Therapy of Desire: Theory and Practice in Hellenistic Ethics.* Princeton University Press.

"be wrong about their health": Martha C Nussbaum (1994). *The Therapy of Desire: Theory and Practice in Hellenistic Ethics.* Princeton University Press.

CHAPTER 7

MEDITATIONS ON DEATH

"Meditate then, on all these things, and on those things which are related to them, both day and night, and both alone and with like-minded companions. For if you will do this, you will never be disturbed while asleep or awake by imagined fears, but you will live like a god among men."

—Epicurus, *Letter to Menoeceus*

Spiritual exercises have been practiced throughout time. They are not related to a particular social structure or to precise conditions. In the same way that performing physical exercises gives athletes new form and strength to their bodies, meditation develops the strength of the mind, transforms the vision of the world, and finally the entire being. As opposed to the Buddhist meditation of the Far East, Epicurean meditation is not associated with the physical body, but it is strictly intellectual and fantastical. In the first place it involves memorizing and assimilating the key tenets of the school that entail an utter adaptation of false popular beliefs: we are to reject the mistaken values of wealth, fame, and power, and strive for the simple and pleasant life. We also become detached from our traditions and social biases, have our view of life reformed, and our outlook of the world is transformed into a natural interpretation. By learning meditation, our perspective of the cosmos will be entirely restructured. The disciple is urged to practice day and night both by himself and with a like-minded friend so that he will never be disturbed either when awake or asleep, and live as a god among men. Especially *the exercise on death*, which takes on a new meaning—it becomes the consciousness of the finitude of existence that gives an infinite value to each moment; the disciple is prompted to regard every new day that dawns to be his last so that he greets each new hour with gratitude.

Meditations on physics, philosophy, friendship, and death constitute the core transformative exercises. It is vital that the meditated phrases are expressed in the most imposing and solid manner. They should consist of a handful of words with a clear and simple meaning, so that they will be easily memorized, accessed, and retrieved during meditation as well as when life's upheavals present themselves. They are to be accepted without hesitation in order to be effective. To avoid confusion and disorientation, questioning and conversation on details are to be allowed only to an advanced disciple.

Meditations on living well and dying well

Meditate telling yourself each day any of the following Epicurean sayings:

Living philosophically

"*The art of living* well and the art of dying well are one."

"*Necessity is an evil*; but there is no necessity for continuing to live with necessity."

"*The spirit looks neither ahead* nor behind. Only the present is our happiness."

"*We must free ourselves* from the prison of public education and politics."

"*The greatest fruit* of self-sufficiency is freedom."

"*Do not spoil* what you have by desiring what you have not."

"*Live unnoticed.*"

"*He who is not satisfied* with a little, is satisfied with nothing."

"*It is better for you* to be free of fear lying upon a pallet, than to have a golden couch and a rich table and be full of trouble."

"*We must laugh* and philosophize and manage our households and look after our other affairs all at the same time, and never stop proclaiming the words of the true philosophy."

"*Every desire must* be confronted by this question: what will happen to me if the object of my desire is accomplished, and what if it is not?"

"*I have never wished* to cater to the crowd; for what I know they do not approve, and what they approve I do not know."

"*The wise man when* he has accommodated himself to straits knows better how to give than to receive, so great is the treasure of self-sufficiency which he has discovered."

"*We must envy no one*; for the good do not deserve envy and as for the bad, the more they prosper, the more they ruin it for themselves."

"*If you fight against* all sensations, you will have no standard by which to judge even those of them which you say are false."

"*All bodily suffering* is easy to disregard: for that which causes acute pain has short duration, and that which endures long in the flesh causes but mild pain."

"*It is easy to commit* an injustice undetected, but impossible to be sure that you have escaped detection."

"*For most people*, to be quiet is to be numb and to be active is to be frenzied."

"*It is not the stomach* that is insatiable, as is generally said, but the false opinion that the stomach needs an unlimited amount to fill it."

"*Frugality too has a limit*, and the man who disregards it is like him who errs through excess."

"Meditate then, on all these things, and on those things which are related to them, both day and night, and both alone and with like-minded companions. For if you will do this, you will never be disturbed while asleep or awake by imagined fears, but you will live like a god among men. For a man who lives among immortal blessings is in no respect like a mortal being."

"Don't fear god; don't worry about death; what is good is easy to get; what is terrible is easy to endure." (tetrapharmakos)

"Empty is that philosopher's argument by which no human suffering is therapeutically treated. For just as there is no use in a medical art that does not cast out the sicknesses of bodies, so too there is no use in philosophy, unless it casts out the suffering of the soul."

Living a pleasant life

"Not what we have but what we enjoy, constitutes our abundance."

"If thou will make a man happy, add not unto his riches but take away from his desires."

"The flesh cries out to be saved from hunger, thirst, and cold. For if a man possesses this safety and hope to possess it, he might rival even Zeus in happiness."

"It is impossible to live a pleasant life without living wisely and well and justly. And it is impossible to live wisely and well and justly without living a pleasant life."

"We must then meditate on the things that make our happiness, seeing that when that is with us, we have all, but when it is absent, we do all to win it."

"He who has learned the limits of life knows that that which removes the pain due to want and makes the whole of life complete is readily procured, so that there is no need of actions which involve struggle."

"Poverty, when measured by the natural purpose of life, is great wealth, but unlimited wealth is great poverty."

"*We should not spoil* what we have by desiring what we do not have, but remember that what we have too was the gift of fortune."

"*We must heal our misfortunes* by the grateful recollection of what has been and by the recognition that it is impossible to undo that which has been done."

"I *have had all the pleasure* I could have expected."

"*We call pleasure the alpha* and omega of a blessed life."

"*By pleasure we mean* the absence of pain in the body and of trouble in the soul."

"*Plain savours bring us a* pleasure equal to a luxurious diet, when all the pain due to want is removed."

"*We have need of pleasure*, when we feel pain owing to the absence of pleasure."

"*the good on certain occasions* we treat as bad, and conversely the bad as good."

"*Bread and water produce* the highest pleasure, when one who needs them puts them to his lips."

"*grow accustomed therefore* to simple and not luxurious diet gives us health to the full, and makes a man alert for the needful employments of life."

"*No pleasure is a bad thing* in itself: but the means which produce some pleasures bring with them disturbances many times greater than the pleasures."

"*Every pleasure because of its natural kinship to us is good*, yet not every pleasure is to be chosen: even as every pain also is an evil, yet not all are always of a nature to be avoided."

"*The limit of quantity in pleasures* is the removal of all that is painful. Wherever pleasure is present, as long as it is there, there is neither pain of body nor of mind, nor of both at once."

"We recognize pleasure as the first good innate in us, and from pleasure we begin every act of choice and avoidance, and to pleasure we return again, using the feeling as the standard by which we judge every good."

"We do not choose every pleasure, but sometimes we pass over many pleasures, when greater discomfort accrues to us as the result of them: and similarly we think many pains better than pleasures, since a greater pleasure comes to us when we have endured pains for some time."

"Pleasure is not an unbroken succession of drinking-bouts and of merrymaking, not sexual love, not the enjoyment of the fish and other delicacies of a luxurious table, which produce a pleasant life; it is sober reasoning, searching out the grounds of every choice and avoidance, and banishing those beliefs through which the greatest disturbances take possession of the soul."

"When we maintain that pleasure is the end, we do not mean the pleasures of profligates and those that consist in sensuality, as is supposed by some who are either ignorant or disagree with us or do not understand, but freedom from pain in the body and from trouble in the mind."

"Infinite time contains no greater pleasure than limited time, if one measures by reason the limits of pleasure."

Infinity of universe

"The universe consists of infinite atoms moving in infinite space."

"We should not think that any other end is served by knowledge of celestial phenomena... than freedom from disturbance."

"A man cannot dispel his fear about the most important matters if he does not know what the nature of the universe is, but suspects the truth of some mythical story. So that without natural science it is not possible to attain our pleasures unalloyed."

"*Since space stretches* far beyond the boundaries of our world, into the infinite, our mind seeks to sound out what lies within this infinity, in which the mind can plunge its gaze at will, and to which the mind's thoughts can soar in free flight."

"*Remember that you are mortal* and that, although having but a limited span of life, you have entered into discussions about nature for all time, and see all things that are and will be and were before."

Wealth of Nature

"*Gratitude is due to blessed Nature* because she has made the necessities of life easy to procure and what is hard to procure unnecessary."

"*The wealth required by Nature* is limited and is easy to produce; but the wealth required by vain ideas extends to infinity."

"*The study of Nature does not create men* who are fond of boasting and chattering or who show off the culture that impresses the many, but rather men who are strong and self-sufficient, and who take pride in their own personal qualities not in those that depend on external circumstances."

"*We must not violate Nature*, but obey her; and we shall obey her if we fulfill those desires that are necessary, and also those that are natural but bring no harm to us, while we must sternly reject those that are harmful."

Dancing with friendship

"*All friendship is desirable* in itself, though it starts from the need of help."

"*Before you look for something to eat* and drink you should look around for companions with whom to eat and drink, for life without a friend is just the gulping of a lion and a wolf."

"*It is not so much our friends'* help that helps us as it is the confidence of their help."

"*Friendship dances around the world* bidding us all to awaken to the recognition of happiness."

"*The noble soul occupies itself* with wisdom and friendship; of these the one is a mortal good, the other immortal."

"*Of all the things which wisdom acquires* to produce the blessedness of the complete life, the greatest is the possession of friendship."

"*He is no friend who is continually asking for help*, nor he who never associates help with friendship. For the former barters kindly feeling for a practical return and the latter destroys the hope of good in the future."

"*The sage does not feel* a greater pain when he is tortured than when his friend is tortured, and would die on his friend's behalf; for if he betrays his friend then the rest of his life would be troubled and disturbed on account of his treachery."

"*Those who grasp after friendship* and those who shrink from it are not worthy of approval; on the other hand, it is necessary to risk some pleasure for the pleasures of friendship."

God makes no trouble for others

"*Don't fear god.*"

"*It is vain to ask of the gods* what a man is capable of supplying for himself."

"*If the gods listened* to the prayers of men, all men would quickly have perished: for they are forever praying for evil against one another."

"The statements of the many about the gods are not conceptions derived from sensation, but false suppositions, according to which the greatest misfortunes befall the wicked and the greatest blessings (the good) by the gift of the gods."

"The blessed and indestructible being of the divine has no concerns of its own, nor does it make trouble for others. It is not affected by feelings of anger or benevolence, because these are found where there is lack of strength."

Symmetry of posthumous and prenatal nonexistence

"Look back, then, at how the stretch of unending time before we are born was nothing to us. Nature, therefore, offers this reflection to us of the future time after our eventual death."

"And just as in the time that went before we felt no pain so when we are no more no doubt there will be nothing to us."

Mortality of existence

"We must carry out each action of our lives as if it were the last."

"The life of folly is empty of gratitude, full of anxiety: it is focused wholly on the future."

"While we are speaking, jealous time has flown; seize today without placing your trust in tomorrow."

"Persuade yourself that each *new day* that dawns will be your last; then you will receive each unexpected hour with gratitude. Recognize all the value of each moment of time which is added on as if it were happening by an incredible stroke of luck."

"We are born once, and cannot be born twice, but for all time must be no more. But you, who are not master of tomorrow, postpone your happiness: life is wasted in procrastination and each one of us dies overwhelmed with cares."

"The thought of death is the same as the consciousness of the finite nature of existence, and it is this which gives an infinite value to each instant."

"Those who call soul incorporeal speak foolishly. For if it were so, it could neither act nor be acted upon. But, as it is, both these properties, you see, plainly belong to soul."

"We must recognize generally that the soul is a corporeal thing, composed of fine particles, dispersed all over the frame."

"When the whole body is broken up, the soul is scattered and has no longer the same powers as before, nor the same notions; hence it does not possess sentience either."

"We must try to make the end of the journey better than the beginning, as long as we are journeying; but when we come to the end, we must be happy and content."

"Every man passes out of life as though he had just been born."

"He is a little man in all respects who has many good reasons for quitting life."

Death is nothingness

"Don't worry about death."

"Become accustomed to the belief that death is nothing to us."

"I was not; I have been; I am not; I do not mind."

"Death is meaningless to the living because they are living, and meaningless to the dead... because they are dead."

"So death, the most terrifying of ills, is nothing to us, since so long as we exist, death is not with us; but when death comes, then we do not exist. It does not then concern either the living or the dead, since for the former it is not, and the latter are no more."

"*Death is nothing to us*, for that which is dissolved is without sensation; and that which lacks sensation is nothing to us."

"*The man speaks but idly* who says that he fears death not because it will be painful when it comes, but because it is painful in anticipation."

"*A right understanding* that death is nothing to us makes the mortality of life enjoyable, not because it adds to it an infinite span of time, but because it takes away the craving for immortality. For there is nothing terrible in life for the man who has truly comprehended that there is nothing terrible in not living."

"*I have anticipated you*, Fortune, and entrenched myself against all your secret attacks. And we will not give ourselves up as captives to you or to any other circumstance; but when it is time for us to go, spitting contempt on life and on those who here vainly cling to it, we will leave life crying aloud in a glorious triumph-song that we have lived well."

References

"the exercise on death": 1. Pierre Hadot (1995). *Philosophy as a Way of Life: Spiritual Exercises from Socrates to Foucault,* translated by Michael Chase.

"The art of living": Epicurus, fragment. See also 1. Fromm, Erich. *The Art of Being.* 2. Fromm, Erich. *The Art of Loving.* 3. Fromm, Erich. *To Have or to Be?*

Necessity is an evil": Vatican Saying 9

"The spirit looks neither ahead": In this verse from Goethe's Second Faust, we find an expression of the art of concentrating on and recognizing the value of the present instant. It corresponds to an experience of time that was lived with particular intensity in the philosophy of Epicurus. See also Pierre Hadot (1995). *Philosophy as a Way of Life: Spiritual Exercises from Socrates to Foucault,* translated by Michael Chase.

We must free ourselves": Vatican Saying 58

"The greatest fruit": Vatican Saying 27

"Do not spoil": Vatican Saying 35

"Live unnoticed." The famous advice of Epicurus lathe biosas, "Live unknown." This saying is not found in the extant writings and is reported by Plutarch invidiously, as if Epicurus had courted fame by his writings while advising his disciples to shun it. See also Norman Wentworth Dewitt (1954). *Epicurus and His Philosophy,* University of Minnesota Press, Minneapolis.

"He who is not satisfied": Vatican Saying 68

"It is better for you": Epicurus, fragment

"We must laugh": Vatican Saying 41

"Every desire must": Vatican Saying 71

"I have never wished": Seneca. *Letters*, Book I – *Letter* XXIX

"The wise man when": Vatican Saying 44

"We must envy no one": Vatican Saying 53

"If you fight against": Principal Doctrine 23

"All bodily suffering": Vatican Saying 4

"It is easy to commit": Vatican Saying 7

"For most people": Vatican Saying 11

"It is not the stomach": Vatican Saying 59

"Frugality too has a limit": Vatican Saying 63

"Meditate then": Epicurus, *Letter to Menoeceus*

"Don't fear god" Tetrapharmakos, The Herculaneum papyri. They consist of more than 1800 papyri found in the Herculaneum Villa of the Papyri, in the 18th century, carbonized by the eruption of Mount Vesuvius in AD 79. The papyri, containing a number of Greek philosophical texts, come from the only surviving library from antiquity that exists in its entirety. Most of the works discovered are associated with the Epicurean philosopher and poet Philodemus of Gadara.

"Empty is that philosopher's": 1. Martha C Nussbaum (1994). *The Therapy of Desire: Theory and Practice in Hellenistic Ethics*. Princeton University Press. 2. Porphyry, Ad Marc. 31, p. 209.

"Not what we have": Epicurean saying

"If thou will make a man happy": Epicurean saying

"The flesh cries out to be saved": Vatican Saying 33

"It is impossible to live": Vatican Saying 5

"We must then meditate": Epicurus, *Letter to Menoeceus*

"He who has learned": Principal doctrine 25

"Poverty, when measured": Vatican Saying 25

"We should not spoil": Vatican Saying 35

"We must heal our misfortunes": Vatican Saying 55

"I have had all the pleasure": Epicurean saying

"We call pleasure the alpha": Epicurus, *Letter to Menoeceus*, Hicks transl.

"By pleasure we mean": Epicurus, *Letter to Menoeceus*

"Plain savours bring us": Epicurus, *Letter to Menoeceus*

"We have need of pleasure": Epicurus, *Letter to Menoeceus*

"The good on certain occasions": Epicurus, *Letter to Menoeceus*

"Bread and water produce": Epicurus, *Letter to Menoeceus*

"Grow accustomed therefore": Epicurus, *Letter to Menoeceus*

"No pleasure is a bad thing": Principal doctrine 8

"Every pleasure because of its natural kinship to us is good": Epicurus, *Letter to Menoeceus*

"The limit of quantity in pleasure": Principal doctrine 3

"We recognize pleasure": Epicurus, *Letter to Menoeceus*

"We do not choose every pleasure": Epicurus, *Letter to Menoeceus*

"Pleasure is not an unbroken succession": Epicurus, *Letter to Menoeceus*

"When we maintain that pleasure": Epicurus, *Letter to Menoeceus*

"Infinite time contains": Principal doctrine 19

"The universe consists of": 1. Lucretius, *On the Nature of Things.* 2. Hawking, Stephen. *A Brief History of Time: From Big Bang to Black Holes.* 3. Hawking, Stephen. *The Theory of Everything: The Origin and Fate of the Universe.* 4. Hawking, Stephen and Mlodinow, Leonard. *The Grand Design.*

"We should not think that": Epicurus, *Letter to Pythocles*

"A man cannot dispel his fear": Principal doctrine 12

"Since space stretches": 1. Lucretius, *On the Nature of Things.* 2. Pierre Hadot (1995*). Philosophy as a Way of Life: Spiritual Exercises from Socrates to Foucault.* Translated by Michael Chase.

"Remember that you are mortal": Vatican Saying 10

"Gratitude is due to blessed Nature": Epicurus, fragment

"The wealth required by Nature": Vatican Saying 65

"The study of Nature does not create men": Vatican Saying 45

"We must not violate Nature": Vatican Saying 21

"All friendship is desirable": Vatican Saying 23

"Before you look for something to eat": Epicurean saying

"It is not so much our friends' ": Vatican Saying 34

"Friendship dances around the world": Vatican Saying 52

"The noble soul occupies itself": Vatican Saying 78

"Of all the things which wisdom acquires": Principal doctrine 27

"He is no friend who is continually asking for help": Vatican Saying 39

"The sage does not feel": Vatican Saying 56–57

"Those who grasp after friendship": Vatican Saying 28

"Don't fear god": expert from Tetrafarmakos

"It is vain to ask of the gods": Vatican Saying 65

"If the gods listened": Epicurus, fragment

"The statements of the many": Epicurus, *Letter to Menoeceus*

"The blessed and indestructible being": Vatican Saying 1

"Look back, then": Lucretius, *On the Nature of Things*.

"And just as in the time": Lucretius, *On the Nature of Things*.

"We must carry out": Pierre Hadot (1995*). Philosophy as a Way of Life: Spiritual Exercises from Socrates to Foucault.* Translated by Michael Chase.

"The life of folly is empty": Seneca*, Letter XV, on Epicurus*

"While we are speaking": Horace. *The Epistles of Horace Ode 1.11.* 2. Horace and Radice Betty. *The Complete Odes and Epodes.*

"Persuade yourself that each new day": 1. Horace. *The Epistles of Horace Ode 1.11.* 2. Horace and Radice Betty. *The Complete Odes and Epodes.* 3. Pierre Hadot (1995). *Philosophy as a Way of Life: Spiritual Exercises from Socrates to Foucault,* translated by Michael Chase.

"We are born once": Vatican Saying 14

"The thought of death": Horace, *Letter,* I, 4, 13-14: "Omnem crede diem tibi diluxisse supremum; gratia superveniet quae non sperabitur hora." Once again, we encounter the Epicurean theme of gratitude. See also Pierre Hadot (1995). *Philosophy as a Way of Life: Spiritual Exercises from Socrates to Foucault.* Translated by Michael Chase.

"Those who call soul incorporeal": Epicurus, *Letter to Herodotus*

"We must recognize": Epicurus, *Letter to Herodotus*

"When the whole body": Epicurus, *Letter to Herodotus*

"We must try to make the end of the journey": Vatican Saying 48

"Every man passes out of life": Vatican Saying 60

"He is a little man in all respects": Vatican Saying 38

"Don't worry about death": expert from Tetrafarmakos

"Become accustomed": Epicurus, *Letter to Menoeceus*

"I was not; I have been; I am not; I do not mind*"*: Epicurean epitaph inscribed on the gravestones of Epicureans and can still be seen on many ancient gravestones of the Roman Empire, and is often used at humanist funerals: Non fui, fui, non sum, non curo (*I was not; I have been*; I am not; I do not mind). This epitaph arose from the doctrine: "Death is nothing to us, for that which is dissolved is without sensation; and that which lacks sensation is nothing to us." (Principal doctrine 2).

"Death is meaningless to the living": Epicurean saying

"So death, the most terrifying of ills": Epicurus, *Letter to Menoeceus*

"Death is nothing to us": Principal doctrine 2

"The man speaks but idly": Epicurus, *Letter to Menoeceus*

"A right understanding": Epicurus, *Letter to Menoeceus*

"I have anticipated you": Vatican Saying 47

CHAPTER 8

EUTHANASIA

"Necessity is an evil; but there is no necessity for continuing to live subject to necessity."

—Epicurus, *Vatican Sayings*

Overcoming the terror of death in no way implies desiring it. We should not expand our view so far that it accommodates an aversion to life and denial of our being. Quite the opposite: we are aware that death eradicates sensation, that senses are essential to pleasure, and pleasure is the ultimate good: therefore, nothing else can be the ultimate purpose of life, but pleasure.

Epicurus is extremely critical about those who are attracted to death, as well as those who are afraid of it. The wise man, Epicurus explains, neither renounces life nor is he afraid of death, since neither living is aggravating or not living is hurtful. Worst of all are those who claim it would have been better *not to be born*, but having been born, the second best outcome is to exit life as soon as possible. And often as a result of the fear of death, such a loathing of life takes hold of human beings that, in their suffering, they take their own life, overlooking that it is fear that is the origin of their pain.

None of us has full ownership of our life, but all have it on lease from Nature. If life is gloomy and carries much more pain than pleasure, why not put an end to it? This is how the philosophical question of logical suicide is brought up. Nature is indifferent to our life and wellbeing. Each of us is the exclusive guardian of his life, thus we have the liberty to end it when the individual deems appropriate. This is the right to autonomy over his life. Autonomy supports his right of self-control and self-respect. It puts forward the question of who owns our life, and an answer would be that naturally, it is the individual himself. Therefore, autonomy maintains that a sane adult has to be allowed to decline medical treatment, for example, even if this could cause his death. It would be heartless and unreasonable to force someone to put up with the intolerable pain against his will. In the event of suffering from a terminal disease or incurable sustained pain, one should have *the sovereignty to opt to end his own life*. Likewise, one should have the choice to bring about his own death with the assistance of a physician, *a procedure known as euthanasia*, or assisted suicide. In most nations, euthanasia is illegal and autonomy is declined; people undergo needless pain because they are not permitted a fast and pain-free death; terminally ill people can be relieved of their suffering if euthanasia is legitimized.

References

"Vatican Sayings": See annex *2*

"not to be born": Epicurus, Letter to Menoeceus

"the sovereignty to opt to end his own life": *Wikipedia, right to die.*

"a procedure known as euthanasia": Wikipedia, *euthanasia*

CHAPTER 9

EPICURUS FACING DEATH

"I have written this letter to you on a happy day to me, which is also the last day of my life. For I have been attacked by a painful inability to urinate, and also dysentery, so violent that nothing can be added to the violence of my sufferings. But the cheerfulness of my mind, which comes from the recollection of all my philosophical contemplation, counterbalances all these afflictions."

—Epicurus, *Letter to Idomeneus*

When facing his death in 270 BC, Epicurus had to stay committed to his own teachings. He could follow one of the two alternatives he used to talk about. The first was to withstand the pain of his illness by recalling the pleasure of the past, and the second was to avoid the suffering by taking his own life. Epicurus chose to withstand his painful illness, showing such courage and tolerance that took both friends and adversaries by surprise. Despite being aware of the fatal outcome of his disease and being subject to unbearable pain, Epicurus used to talk to those visiting him about the usual issues of the time and the nature of things, rather than his illness and suffering. He did his utmost to remain even-tempered, not in need of help or pity. He cherished the pursuit of happiness to the end. To the last moment of his life, he wanted to look and feel happy by practicing his teaching that one could overcome pain and even be joyful by recalling memories of the pleasure of the past. This obsession has its admirers. There is something magnificent in this passion of triumph over pain, in this invocation of the past to compensate for the pain of the present, in this desperate search for happiness despite the manifestation of death. It is not always easy to convince ourselves that we are happy. It demands unquestionable willpower to sustain it. Epicurus was able to realize for himself the utopia of happiness he dreamed of.

He died with his mind attuned to the existence that was deserting him, visualizing his past life to confront the approach of death. The last image of the life that was about to disappear crossed his mind for the final time. He accepted it with gratitude, without regret, without hope. Then, all at once, everything was lost—the present, the past, the future retreating into eternal non-existence.

Sustaining independence and courage in the face of death, when every superstition has been removed, was a truly original attitude that was attributed to Epicurus. He recognized death without terror and without hope. He demonstrated that death could limit life without disturbing it.

References

"Letter to Idomeneus": "I have written this letter to you on a happy day to me, which is also the last day of my life. For I have been attacked by a painful inability to urinate, and also dysentery, so violent that nothing can be added to the violence of my sufferings. But the cheerfulness of my mind, which comes from the recollection of all my philosophical contemplation, counterbalances all these afflictions. And I beg you to take care of the children of Metrodorus, in a manner worthy of the devotion shown by the young man to me, and to philosophy."

ANNEXES

ANNEX 1

THE PRINCIPAL DOCTRINES OF EPICURUS

Translated by Cyril Bailey—Oxford, 1926

1. The blessed and immortal nature knows no trouble itself nor causes trouble to any other, so that it is never constrained by anger or favour. For all such things exist only in the weak.

2. Death is nothing to us, for that which is dissolved is without sensation; and that which lacks sensation is nothing to us.

3. The limit of quantity in pleasures is the removal of all that is painful. Wherever pleasure is present, as long as it is there, there is neither pain of body nor of mind, nor of both at once.

4. Pain does not last continuously in the flesh, but the acutest pain is there for a very short time, and even that which just exceeds the pleasure in the flesh does not continue for many days at once. But chronic illnesses permit a predominance of pleasure over pain in the flesh.

5. It is not possible to live pleasantly without living prudently and honorably and justly, [nor again to live a life of prudence, honor, and Justice] without living pleasantly. And the man who does not possess the pleasant life, is not living prudently and honorably and justly, [and the man who does not possess the virtuous life], cannot possibly live pleasantly.

6. To secure protection from men, anything is a natural good by which you may be able to attain this end.

7. Some men wished to become famous and conspicuous, thinking that they would thus win for themselves safety from other men. Wherefore if the life of such men is safe, they have obtained the good which nature craves; but if it is not safe, they do not possess that for which they strove at first by the instinct of nature.

8. No pleasure is a bad thing in itself: but the means which produce some pleasures bring with them disturbances many times greater than the pleasures.

9. If every pleasure could be intensified so that it lasted and influenced the whole organism or the most essential parts of our nature, pleasures would never differ from one another.

10. If the things that produce the pleasures of profligates could dispel the fears of the mind about the phenomena of the sky and death and its pains, and also teach the limits of desires [and of pains], we should never have cause to blame them: for they would be filling themselves full with pleasures from every source and never have pain of body or mind, which is the evil of life.

11. If we were not troubled by our suspicions of the phenomena of the sky and about death, fearing that it concerns us, and also by our failure to grasp the limits of pains and desires, we should have no need of natural science.

12. A man cannot dispel his fear about the most important matters if he does not know what the nature of the universe is, but suspects the truth of some mythical story. So that without natural science it is not possible to attain our pleasures unalloyed.

13. There is no profit in securing protection in relation to men, if things above and things beneath the Earth and indeed all in the boundless universe remain matters of suspicion.

14. the most unalloyed source of protection from men, which is secured to some extent by a certain force of expulsion, is in fact the immunity which results from a quiet life and the retirement from the world.

15. The wealth demanded by nature is both limited and easily procured; that demanded by idle imaginings stretches on to infinity.

16. In but few things chance hinders a wise man, but the greatest and most important matters reason has ordained and throughout the whole period of life does and will ordain.

17. The just man is most free from trouble, the unjust most full of trouble.

18. The pleasure in the flesh is not increased, when once the pain due to want is removed, but is only varied: and the limit as regards pleasure in the mind is begotten by the reasoned understanding of these very pleasures and of the emotions akin to them, which used to cause the greatest fear to the mind.

19. Infinite time contains no greater pleasure than limited time, if one measures by reason the limits of pleasure.

20. The flesh perceives the limits of pleasure as unlimited, and unlimited time is required to supply it. But the mind, having attained a reasoned understanding of the ultimate good of the flesh and its limits and having dissipated the fears concerning the time to come, supplies us with the complete life, and we have no further need of infinite time: but neither does the mind shun pleasure, nor, when circumstances begin to bring about the departure from life, does it approach its end as though it fell short in any way of the best life.

21. He who has learned the limits of life knows that that which removes the pain due to want and makes the whole of life complete is readily procured, so that there is no need of actions which involve competition.

22. We must consider both the real purpose and all the evidence of direct perception, to which we always refer the conclusions of opinion; otherwise, all will be full of doubt and confusion.

23. If you fight against all sensations, you will have no standard by which to judge even those of them which you say are false.

24. If you reject any single sensation and fail to distinguish between the conclusion of opinion as to the appearance awaiting confirmation and that which is actually given by the sensation or feeling, or each intuitive apprehension of the mind, you will confound all other sensations as well with the same groundless opinion, so that you will reject every standard of judgment. And if among the mental images created by your opinion you affirm both that which awaits confirmation and that which does not, you will not escape error; since you will have preserved the whole cause of doubt in every judgment between what is right and what is wrong.

25. If on each occasion, instead of referring your actions to the end of nature, you turn to some other nearer standard when you are making a choice or an avoidance, your actions will not be consistent with your principles.

26. Of desires, all that do not lead to a sense of pain, if they are not satisfied, are not necessary, but involve a craving which is easily dispelled, when the object is hard to procure or they seem likely to produce harm.

27. Of all the things which wisdom acquires to produce the blessedness of the complete life, far the greatest is the possession of friendship.

28. The same conviction which has given us confidence that there is nothing terrible that lasts forever or even for long, has also seen the protection of friendship most fully completed in the limited evils of this life.

29. Among desires, some are natural [and necessary, some natural] but not necessary, and others neither natural nor necessary, but due to idle imagination.

30. Wherever in the case of desires which are physical, but do not lead to a sense of pain, if they are not fulfilled, the effort is intense, such pleasures are due to idle imagination, and it is not owing to their own nature that they fail to be dispelled, but owing to the empty imaginings of the man.

31. The justice which arises from nature is a pledge of mutual advantage to restrain men from harming one another and save them from being harmed.

32. For all living things which have not been able to make compacts not to harm one another or be harmed, nothing ever is either just or unjust; and likewise too for all tribes of men which have been unable or unwilling to make compacts not to harm or be harmed.

33. Justice never is anything in itself, but in the dealings of men with one another in any place whatever and at any time it is a kind of compact not to harm or be harmed.

34. Injustice is not an evil in itself, but only in consequence of the fear which attaches to the apprehension of being unable to escape those appointed to punish such actions.

35. It is not possible for one who acts in secret contravention of the terms of the compact not to harm or be harmed, to be confident that he will escape detection, even if at present he escapes a thousand times. For up to the time of death it cannot be certain that he will indeed escape.

36. In its general aspect justice is the same for all, for it is a kind of mutual advantage in the dealings of men with one another: but with reference to the individual peculiarities of a country or any other circumstances, the same thing does not turn out to be just for all.

37. Among actions which are sanctioned as just by law, that which is proved on examination to be of advantage in the requirements of men's dealings with one another, has the guarantee of justice, whether it is the same for all or not. But if a man makes a law and it does not turn out to lead to advantage in men's dealings with each other, then it no longer has the essential nature of justice. And even if the advantage in the matter of justice shifts from one side to the other, but for a while accords with the general concept, it is nonetheless just for that period in the eyes of those who do not confound themselves with empty sounds but look to the actual facts.

38. Where, provided the circumstances have not been altered, actions which were considered just, have been shown not to accord with the general concept in actual practice, then they are not just. But where, when circumstances have changed, the same actions which were sanctioned as just no longer lead to advantage, there they were just at the time when they were of advantage for the dealings of fellow-citizens with one another, but subsequently they are no longer just, when no longer of advantage.

39. The man who has best ordered the element of disquiet arising from external circumstances has made those things that he could akin to himself and the rest at least not alien;

but with all to which he could not do even this, he has refrained from mixing, and has expelled from his life all which it was of advantage to treat thus.

40. As many as possess the power to procure complete immunity from their neighbors, these also live most pleasantly with one another, since they have the most certain pledge of security, and after they have enjoyed the fullest intimacy, they do not lament the previous departure of a dead friend, as though he were to be pitied.

ANNEX 2

THE VATICAN SAYINGS

Translated by Cyril Bailey—Oxford, 1926

This list by an unknown author was discovered in 1888 at the Vatican and is reputed to date from the fourteenth century.

1. A blessed and indestructible being has no trouble himself and brings no trouble upon any other being; so he is free from anger and partiality, for all such things imply weakness.

2. Death is nothing to us; for that which has been dissolved into its elements experiences no sensations, and that which has no sensation is nothing to us.

3. Continuous bodily pain does not last long; instead, pain, if extreme, is present a very short time, and even that degree of pain which slightly exceeds bodily pleasure does not last for many days at once. Diseases of long duration allow an excess of bodily pleasure over pain.

4. All bodily suffering is easy to disregard: for that which causes acute pain has short duration, and that which endures long in the flesh causes but mild pain.

5. It is impossible to live a pleasant life without living wisely and honorably and justly, and it is impossible to live wisely and honorably and justly without living pleasantly. Whenever any one of these is lacking, when, for instance, the man is not able to live wisely, though he lives honorably and justly, it is impossible for him to live a pleasant life.

6. It is impossible for a man who secretly violates the terms of the agreement not to harm or be harmed to feel confident that he will remain undiscovered, even if he has already escaped ten thousand times; for until his death he is never sure that he will not be detected. [See Principle Doctrine 35]

7. It is easy to commit an injustice undetected, but impossible to be sure that you have escaped detection.

8. The wealth required by nature is limited and is easy to procure; but the wealth required by vain ideals extends to infinity. [See Principle Doctrine 15]

9. Necessity is an evil, but there is no necessity to live under the control of necessity.

10. Remember that you are mortal and have a limited time to live and have devoted yourself to discussions on Nature for all time and eternity and have seen things that are now and are to come and have been.

11. For most people, to be quiet is to be numb and to be active is to be frenzied.

12. The just man is most free from disturbance, while the unjust is full of the utmost disturbance. [See Principle Doctrine 17]

13. Among the things held to be just by law, whatever is proved to be of advantage in men's dealings has the stamp of justice, whether or not it be the same for all; but if a man makes a law and it does not prove to be mutually advantageous, then this is no longer just. And if what is mutually advantageous varies and only for a time corresponds to our concept of justice, nevertheless for that time it is just for those who do not trouble themselves about empty words, but look simply at the facts. [See Principle Doctrine 37]

14. We are born once and cannot be born twice, but for all time must be no more. But you, who are not master of tomorrow, postpone your happiness. Life is wasted in procrastination, and each one of us dies without allowing himself leisure.

15. We value our characters as something peculiar to ourselves, whether they are good and we are esteemed by men or not, so ought we to value the characters of others, if they are well-disposed to us.

16. No one when he sees evil deliberately chooses it, but is enticed by it as being good in comparison with a greater evil and so pursues it.

17. It is not the young man who should be thought happy, but the old man who has lived a good life. For the young man at the height of his powers is unstable and is carried this way and that by fortune, like a headlong stream. But the old man has come to anchor in old age as though in port, and the good things for which before he hardly hoped he has brought into safe harbor in his grateful recollections.

18. If sight, association, and intercourse are removed, the passion of love is ended.

19. Forgetting the good that has been, he has become old this very day.

20. Of our desires some are natural and necessary, others are natural but not necessary; and others are neither natural nor necessary, but are due to groundless opinion. [See Principle Doctrine 29]

21. We must not violate nature, but obey her; and we shall obey her if we fulfill those desires that are necessary, and also those that are natural but bring no harm to us, but we must sternly reject those that are harmful.

22. Unlimited time and limited time afford an equal amount of pleasure, if we measure the limits of that pleasure by reason. [See Principle Doctrine 19]

23. All friendship is desirable in itself, though it starts from the need of help.

24. Dreams have neither divine character nor any prophetic force, but they originate from the influx of images.

25. Poverty, when measured by the natural purpose of life, is great wealth, but unlimited wealth is great poverty.

26. You must understand that whether the discourse is long or short it tends to the same end.

27. In all other occupations the fruit comes painfully after completion, but in philosophy pleasure goes hand in hand with knowledge; for enjoyment does not follow comprehension, but comprehension and enjoyment are simultaneous.

28. We must not approve either those who are always ready for friendship, or those who hang back, but for friendship's sake we must run risks.

29. In investigating nature I would prefer to speak openly and like an oracle to give answers serviceable to all mankind, even though no one should understand me, rather than to conform to popular opinions and so win the praise freely scattered by the mob.

30. Some men throughout their lives spend their time gathering together the means of life, for they do not see that the draught swallowed by all of us at birth is a draught of death.

31. Against all else it is possible to provide security, but as against death all of us mortals alike dwell in an unfortified city.

32. The veneration of the wise man is a great blessing to those who venerate him.

33. The flesh cries out to be saved from hunger, thirst, and cold. For if a man possess this safety and hope to possess it, he might rival even Zeus in happiness.

34. It is not so much our friends' help that helps us as it is the confidence of their help.

35. We should not spoil what we have by desiring what we do not have, but remember that what we have too was the gift of fortune.

36. Epicurus' life, when compared to other men's in respect of gentleness and self-sufficiency, might be thought a mere legend.

37. Nature is weak toward evil, not toward good: because it is saved by pleasures, but destroyed by pains.

38. He is a little man in all respects who has many good reasons for quitting life.

39. He is no friend who is continually asking for help, nor he who never associates help with friendship. For the former barters kindly feeling for a practical return and the latter destroys the hope of good in the future.

40. The man who says that all things come to pass by necessity cannot criticize one who denies that all things come to pass by necessity: for he admits that this too happens of necessity.

41. We must laugh and philosophize at the same time and do our household duties and employ our other faculties, and never cease proclaiming the sayings of the true philosophy.

42. The same span of time embraces both the beginning and the end of the greatest good.

43. The love of money, if unjustly gained, is impious, and, if justly gained, is shameful; for it is unseemly to be parsimonious even with justice on one's side.

44. The wise man when he has accommodated himself to straits knows better how to give than to receive, so great is the treasure of self-sufficiency which he has discovered.

45. The study of nature does not make men productive of boasting or bragging nor apt to display that culture which is the object of rivalry with the many, but high-spirited and self-sufficient, taking pride in the good things of their own minds and not of their circumstances.

46. Let us utterly drive from us our bad habits as if they were evil men who have long done us great harm.

47. I have anticipated thee, Fortune, and entrenched myself against all thy secret attacks. And I will not give myself up as captive to thee or to any other circumstance; but when it is time for me to go, spitting contempt on life and on those who vainly cling to it, I will leave life crying aloud a glorious triumph-song that I have lived well.

48. We must try to make the end of the journey better than the beginning, as long as we are journeying; but when we come to the end, we must be happy and content.

49. It is impossible for someone to dispel his fears about the most important matters if he does not know the nature of the universe but still gives some credence to myths. So without the study of Nature there is no enjoyment of pure pleasure. [See Principle Doctrine 12]

50. No pleasure is a bad thing in itself, but the things which produce certain pleasures entail disturbances many times greater than the pleasures themselves. [See Principle Doctrine 8]

51. You tell me that the stimulus of the flesh makes you too prone to the pleasures of love. Provided that you do not break the laws or good customs and do not distress any of your neighbors or do harm to your body or squander your pittance, you may indulge your inclination as you please. Yet it is

impossible not to come up against one or other of these barriers, for the pleasures of love never profited a man and he is lucky if they do him no harm.

52. Friendship dances around the world bidding us all to awaken to the recognition of happiness.

53. We must envy no one, for the good do not deserve envy and the bad, the more they prosper, the more they injure themselves.

54. We must not pretend to study philosophy, but study it in reality, for it is not the appearance of health that we need, but real health.

55. We must heal our misfortunes by the grateful recollection of what has been and by the recognition that it is impossible to undo that which has been done.

56. The wise man feels no more pain when being tortured himself than when his friend tortured.

57. On occasion a man will die for his friend, for if he betrays his friend, his whole life will be confounded by distrust and completely upset.

58. We must free ourselves from the prison of public education and politics.

59. It is not the stomach that is insatiable, as is generally said, but the false opinion that the stomach needs an unlimited amount to fill it.

60. Every man passes out of life as though he had just been born.

61. Most beautiful too is the sight of those near and dear to us, when our original kinship makes us of one mind; for such sight is great incitement to this end.

62. Now if parents are justly angry with their children, it is certainly useless to fight against it and not to ask for pardon; but if their anger is unjust and irrational, it is quite ridiculous to add fuel to their irrational passion by nursing one's own indignation, and not to attempt to turn aside their wrath in other ways by gentleness.

63. Frugality too has a limit, and the man who disregards it is like him who errs through excess.

64. Praise from others must come unasked, and we must concern ourselves with the healing of our own lives.

65. It is vain to ask of the gods what a man is capable of supplying for himself.

66. Let us show our feeling *for our lost friends* not by lamentation but by meditation.

67. A free life cannot acquire many possessions, because this is not easy to do without servility to mobs or monarchs, yet it possesses all things in unfailing abundance; and if by chance it obtains many possessions, it is easy to distribute them so as to win the gratitude of neighbors.

68. Nothing is sufficient for him to whom what is sufficient seems too little.

69. The ungrateful greed of the soul makes the creature everlastingly desire varieties in its lifestyle.

70. Let nothing be done in your life which will because you fear if it becomes known to your neighbor.

71. Every desire must be confronted by this question: what will happen to me if the object of my desire is accomplished, and what if it is not?

72. There is no advantage to obtaining protection from other men so long as we are alarmed by events above or below the Earth or in general by whatever happens in the boundless universe.

73. The occurrence of certain bodily pains assists us in guarding against others like them.

74. In a philosophical discussion, he who is defeated gains more, since he learns more.

75. The saying, "look to the end of a long life," shows ungratefulness for past good fortune.

76. You are in your old age just such as I urge you to be, and you have seen the difference between studying philosophy for oneself and proclaiming it to Greece at large; I rejoice with you.

77. The greatest fruit of self-sufficiency is freedom.

78. The noble soul occupies itself with wisdom and friendship; of these the one is a mortal good, the other immortal.

79. The man who is serene causes no disturbance to himself or to another.

80. The first measure of security is to watch over one's youth and to guard against what makes havoc of all by means of maddening desires.

81. The disturbance of the soul cannot be ended nor true joy created either by the possession of the greatest wealth or by honor and respect in the eyes of the mob or by anything else that is associated with or caused by unlimited desire.

ANNEX 3

THE LETTER OF EPICURUS TO MENOECEUS

Translated by Cyril Bailey—Oxford, 1926

Greeting,

Let no one when young delay to study philosophy, nor when he is old grow weary of his study. For no one can come too early or too late to secure the health of his soul. And the man who says that the age for philosophy has either not yet come or has gone by is like the man who says that the age for happiness is not yet come to him, or has passed away. Wherefore, both when young and old, a man must study philosophy, so that as he grows old he may be young in blessings through the grateful recollection of what has been, and in youth he may be old as well, since he will know no fear of what is to come. We must then meditate on the things that make our happiness, seeing that when that is with us, we have all, but when it is absent, we do all to win it.

The things which I used unceasingly to commend to you, these, do and practice, considering them to be the first principles of the good life. First of all, believe that god is a being immortal and blessed, even as the common idea of a god is engraved on men's minds, and do not assign to him anything alien to his immortality or ill-suited to his blessed-ness: but believe about him everything that can uphold his blessedness and immortality. For gods there are, since the knowledge of them is by clear vision. But they are not such as the many believe them to be: for indeed they do not consistently represent them as they believe them to be. And the impious man is not he who popularly denies the gods of the many, but he who attaches to the gods the beliefs of the many. For the statements of the many about the gods are not conceptions derived from sensation, but false suppositions, according to which the greatest misfortunes befall the wicked and the greatest blessings (the good) by the gift of the gods. For men, being accustomed always to their own virtues, welcome those like themselves, but regard all that is not of their nature as alien.

Become accustomed to the belief that death is nothing to us. For all good and evil consists of sensation, but death is deprivation of sensation. And therefore, a right understanding that death is nothing to us makes the mortality of life enjoyable, not because it adds to it an infinite span of time, but because it takes away the craving for immortality.

For there is nothing terrible in life for the man who has truly comprehended that there is nothing terrible in not living. So that the man speaks but idly who says that he fears death not because it will be painful when it comes, but because it is painful in anticipation. For that which gives no trouble when it comes is but an empty pain in anticipation. So death, the most terrifying of ills, is nothing to us, since so long as we exist, death is not with us; but when death comes, then we do not exist. It does not then concern either the living or the dead, since for the former it is not, and the latter are no more.

But the many at one moment shun death as the greatest of evils, at another, [yearn for it] as a respite from the [evils] in life. But the wise man neither seeks to escape life nor fears the cessation of life, for neither does life offend him nor does the absence of life seem to be any evil. And just as with food, he does not seek simply the larger share and nothing else, but rather the most pleasant, so he seeks to enjoy not the longest period of time, but the most pleasant. And he who counsels the young man to live well, but the old man to make a good end, is foolish, not merely because of the desirability of life, but also because it is the same training which teaches to live well and to die well. Yet much worse still is the man who says it is good not to be born but once born makes haste to pass the gates of Death. For if he says this from conviction why does he not pass away out of life? For it is open to him to do so, if he had firmly made up his mind to this. But if he speaks in jest, his words are idle among men who cannot receive them.

We must then bear in mind that the future is neither ours, nor yet wholly not ours, so that we may not altogether expect it as sure to come, nor abandon hope of it, as if it will certainly not come.

We must consider that of desires, some are natural, others vain; and of the natural, some are necessary and others merely natural; and of the necessary, some are necessary for happiness, others for the repose of the body, and others for very life. The right understanding of these facts enables us to refer all choice and avoidance to the health of the body and [the soul's] freedom from disturbance, since this is the aim of the life of blessedness. For it is to obtain this end that we always act, namely, to avoid pain and fear. And when this is once secured for us, all the tempest of the soul is dispersed, since the living creature has not to wander as though in search of something that is missing, and to look for some other thing by which he can fulfill the good of the soul and the good of the body. For it is then that we have need of pleasure, when we feel pain owing to the absence of pleasure; [but when we do not feel pain], we no longer need pleasure. And for this cause we call pleasure the beginning and end of the blessed life. For we recognize pleasure as the first good innate in us, and from pleasure we begin every act of choice and avoidance, and to pleasure we return again, using the feeling as the standard by which we judge every good.

And since pleasure is the first good and natural to us, for this very reason we do not choose every pleasure, but sometimes we pass over many pleasures, when greater discomfort accrues to us as the result of them: and similarly we think many pains better than pleasures, since a greater pleasure comes to us when we have endured pains for a long time. Every pleasure then because of its natural kinship to us is good, yet not every pleasure is to be chosen: even as every pain also is an evil, yet not all are always of a nature to be avoided. Yet by a scale of comparison and by the consideration of advantages and disadvantages we must form our judgment on all these matters. For the good on certain occasions we treat as bad, and conversely the bad as good.

And again independence of desire we think a great good— not that we may at all times enjoy but a few things, but that, if we do not possess many, we may enjoy the few in the genuine persuasion that those have the sweetest pleasure in luxury who least need it, and that all that is natural is easy to be obtained, but that which is superfluous is hard. And so plain savours bring us a pleasure equal to a luxurious diet, when all the pain due to want is removed; and bread and water produce the highest pleasure, when one who needs them puts them to his lips. To grow accustomed therefore to simple and not luxurious diet gives us health to the full, and makes a man alert for the needful employments of life, and when after long intervals we approach luxuries disposes us better towards them, and fits us to be fearless of fortune.

When, therefore, we maintain that pleasure is the end, we do not mean the pleasures of profligates and those that consist in sensuality, as is supposed by some who are either ignorant or disagree with us or do not understand, but freedom from pain in the body and from trouble in the mind. For it is not continuous drinkings and revelings, nor the satisfaction of lusts, nor the enjoyment of fish and other luxuries of the wealthy table, which produce a pleasant life, but sober reasoning, searching out the motives for all choice and avoidance, and banishing mere opinions, to which are due the greatest disturbance of the spirit.

Of all this, the beginning and the greatest good is prudence. Wherefore prudence is a more precious thing even than philosophy: for from prudence are sprung all the other virtues, and it teaches us that it is not possible to live pleasantly without living prudently and honourably and justly, [nor, again, to live a life of prudence, honour, and justice] without living pleasantly. For the virtues are by nature bound up with the pleasant life, and the pleasant life is inseparable from them. For indeed, who, think you, is a better man than he who holds reverent opinions concerning the gods, and is at all times free from fear of death, and has reasoned out the end ordained by nature? He understands that the limit of good things is easy to fulfill and easy to attain, whereas the course of ills is either short in time or slight in pain; he laughs at [destiny], whom some have introduced as the mistress of all things. [He thinks that with us lies the chief power in determining events, some of which happen by necessity] and some by chance, and some are within our control; for while necessity cannot be called to account, he sees that chance is inconstant, but that which is in our control is subject to no master, and to it are naturally attached praise and blame. For, indeed, it was better to follow the myths about the gods than to become a slave to the destiny of the natural philosophers: for the former suggests a hope of placating the gods by worship, whereas the latter involves a necessity which knows no placation. As to chance, he does not regard it as a god as most men do [for in a god's acts there is no disorder], nor as an uncertain cause [of all things] for he does not believe that good and evil are given by chance to man for the framing of a blessed life, but that opportunities for great good and great evil are afforded by it. He therefore thinks it better to be unfortunate in reasonable action than to prosper in unreason. For it is better in a man's actions that what is well-chosen [should fail, rather than that what is ill chosen] should be successful owing to chance.

Meditate, therefore, on these things, and things akin to them, night and day by yourself; and with a companion like to yourself, and never shall you be disturbed waking or asleep, but you shall live like a god among men. For a man who lives among immortal blessings is not like unto a mortal being.

ANNEX 4

THE LETTER OF EPICURUS TO HERODOTUS

Translated by Robert Drew Hicks, 1925

For those who are unable to study carefully all my physical writings or to go into the longer treatises at all, I have myself prepared an epitome of the whole system, Herodotus, to preserve in the memory enough of the principal doctrines, to the end that on every occasion they may be able to aid themselves on the most important points, so far as they take up the study of Physics. Those who have made some advance in the survey of the entire system ought to fix in their minds under the principal headings an elementary outline of the whole treatment of the subject. For a comprehensive view is often required, the details but seldom.

To the former, then—the main heads—we must continually return, and must memorize them so far as to get a valid conception of the facts, as well as the means of discovering all the details exactly when once the general outlines are rightly understood and remembered; since it is the privilege of the mature student to make a ready use of his conceptions by referring every one of them to elementary facts and simple terms. For it is impossible to gather up the results of continuous diligent study of the entirety of things, unless we can embrace in short formulas and hold in mind all that might have been accurately expressed even to the minutest detail.

Hence, since such a course is of service to all who take up natural science, I, who devote to the subject my continuous energy and reap the calm enjoyment of a life like this, have prepared for you just such an epitome and manual of the doctrines as a whole.

In the first place, Herodotus, you must understand what it is that words denote, in order that by reference to this we may be in a position to test opinions, inquiries, or problems, so that our proofs may not run on untested ad infinitum, nor the terms we use be empty of meaning. For the primary signification of every term employed must be clearly seen, and ought to need no proving; this being necessary, if we are to have something to which the point at issue or the problem or the opinion before us can be referred.

Next, we must by all means stick to our sensations, that is, simply to the present impressions whether of the mind or of any criterion whatever, and similarly to our actual feelings, in order that we may have the means of determining that which needs confirmation and that which is obscure.

When this is clearly understood, it is time to consider generally things which are obscure. To begin with, nothing comes into being out of what is non-existent. For in that case anything would have arisen out of anything, standing as it would in no need of its proper germs. And if that which disappears had been destroyed and become non-existent, everything would have perished, that into which the things were dissolved being non-existent. Moreover, the sum total of things was always such as it is now, and such it will ever remain. For there is nothing into which it can change. For outside the sum of things there is nothing which could enter into it and bring about the change.

Further, the whole of being consists of bodies and space. For the existence of bodies is everywhere attested by sense itself, and it is upon sensation that reason must rely when it attempts to infer the unknown from the known. And if there were no space (which we call also void and place and intangible nature), bodies would have nothing in which to be and through which to move, as they are plainly seen to move. Beyond bodies and space there is nothing which by mental apprehension or on its analogy we can conceive to exist. When we speak of bodies and space, both are regarded as wholes or separate things, not as the properties or accidents of separate things.

Again, of bodies some are composite, others the elements of which these composite bodies are made. These elements are indivisible and unchangeable, and necessarily so, if things are not all to be destroyed and pass into non-existence, but are to be strong enough to endure when the composite bodies are broken up, because they possess, a solid nature and are incapable of being anywhere or anyhow dissolved. It follows that the first beginnings must be indivisible, corporeal entities.

Again, the sum of things is infinite. For what is finite has an extremity, and the extremity of anything is discerned only by comparison with something else. Now the sum of things is not discerned by comparison with anything else: hence it has no extremity, it has no limit; and, since it has no limit, it must be unlimited or infinite.

Moreover, the sum of things is unlimited both by reason of the multitude of the atoms and the extent of the void. For if the void were infinite and bodies finite, the bodies would not have stayed anywhere but would have been dispersed in their course through the infinite void, not having any supports or counter-checks to send them back on their upward rebound. Again, if the void were finite, the infinity of bodies would not have anywhere to be.

Furthermore, the atoms, which have no void in them—out of which composite bodies arise and into which they are dissolved—vary indefinitely in their shapes; for so many varieties of things as we see could never have arisen out of a recurrence of a definite number of the same shapes. The like atoms of each shape are absolutely infinite; but the variety of shapes, though indefinitely large, is not absolutely infinite.

The atoms are in continual motion through all eternity. Some of them rebound to a considerable distance from each other, while others merely oscillate in one place when they chance to have got entangled or to be enclosed by a mass of other atoms shaped for entangling.

This is because each atom is separated from the rest by void, which is incapable of offering any resistance to the rebound; while it is the solidity of the atom which makes it rebound after a collision, however short the distance to which it rebounds, when it finds itself imprisoned in a mass of entangling atoms. Of all this there is no beginning, since both atoms and void exist from everlasting.

The repetition at such length of all that we are now re-calling to mind furnishes an adequate outline for our conception of the nature of things.

Moreover, there is an infinite number of worlds, some like this world, and others unlike it. For the atoms being infinite in number, as has just been proved, are borne ever further in their course. For the atoms out of which a world might arise, or by which a world might be formed, have not all been expended on one world or a finite number of worlds, whether like or unlike this one. Hence there will be nothing to hinder an infinity of worlds.

Again, there are outlines or films, which are of the same shape as solid bodies, but of a thinness far exceeding that of any object that we see. For it is not impossible that there should be found in the surrounding air combinations of this kind, materials adapted for expressing the hollowness and thinness of surfaces, and effluxes preserving the same relative position and motion which they had in the solid objects from which they come. To these films we give the name of "images" or "idols." Furthermore, so long as nothing comes in the way to offer resistance, motion through the void accomplishes any imaginable distance in an inconceivably short time. For resistance encountered is the equivalent of slowness, its absence the equivalent of speed.

Not that, if we consider the minute times perceptible by reason alone, the moving body itself arrives at more than one place simultaneously (for this too is inconceivable), although in time perceptible to sense it does arrive simultaneously, however different the point of departure from that conceived by us. For if it changed its direction that would be equivalent to its meeting with resistance, even if up to that point we allow nothing to impede the rate of its flight. This is an elementary fact which in itself is well worth bearing in mind. In the next place the exceeding thinness of the images is contradicted by none of the facts under our observation. Hence also their velocities are enormous, since they always find a void passage to fit them. Besides, their incessant effluence meets with no resistance or very little, although many atoms, not to say an unlimited number, do at once encounter resistance.

Besides this, remember that the production of the images is as quick as thought. For particles are continually streaming off from the surface of bodies, though no diminution of the bodies is observed, because other particles take their place. And those given off for a long time retain the position and arrangement which their atoms had when they formed part of the solid bodies, although occasionally they are thrown into confusion. Sometimes such films a are formed very rapidly in the air, because they need not have any solid content; and there are other modes in which they may be formed. For there is nothing in all this which is contradicted by sensation, if we in some sort look at the clear evidence of sense, to which we should also refer the continuity of particles in the objects external to ourselves.

We must also consider that it is by the entrance of something coming from external objects that we see their shapes and think of them. For external things would not stamp on us their own nature of color and form through the medium of the air which is between them and use or by means of rays of light or currents of any sort going from us to them, so well as by the entrance into our eyes or minds, to whichever their size is suitable, of certain films coming from the things themselves, these films or outlines being of the same color and shape as the external things themselves. They move with rapid motion; and this again explains why they present the appearance of the single continuous object, and retain the mutual interconnection which they had in the object, when they impinge upon the sense, such impact being due to the oscillation of the atoms in the interior of the solid object from which they come. And whatever presentation we derive by direct contact, whether it be with the mind or with the sense-organs, be it shape that is presented or other properties, this shape as presented is the shape of the solid thing, and it is due either to a close coherence of the image as a whole or to a mere remnant of its parts. Falsehood and error always depend upon the intrusion of opinion when a fact awaits confirmation or the absence of contradiction, which fact is afterwards frequently not confirmed or even contradicted following a certain movement in ourselves connected with, but distinct from, the mental picture presented—which is the cause of error.

For the presentations which, for example, are received in a picture or arise in dreams, or from any other form of apprehension by the mind or by the other criteria of truth, would never have resembled what we call the real and true things, had it not been for certain actual things of the kind with which we come in contact. Error would not have occurred, if we had not experienced some other movement in ourselves, conjoined with, but distinct from, the perception of what is presented. And from this movement, if it be not confirmed or be contradicted, falsehood results; while, if it be confirmed or not contradicted, truth results.

And to this view we must closely adhere, if we are not to repudiate the criteria founded on the clear evidence of sense, nor again to throw all these things into confusion by maintaining falsehood as if it were truth.

Again, hearing takes place when a current passes from the object, whether person or thing, which emits voice or sound or noise, or produces the sensation of hearing in any way whatever. This current is broken up into homogeneous particles, which at the same time preserve a certain mutual connection and a distinctive unity extending to the object which emitted them, and thus, for the most part, cause the perception in that case or, if not, merely indicate the presence of the external object. For without the transmission from the object of a certain interconnection of the parts no such sensation could arise. Therefore we must not suppose that the air itself is molded into shape by the voice emitted or something similar; for it is very far from being the case that the air is acted upon by it in this way. The blow which is struck in us when we utter a sound causes such a displacement of the particles as serves to produce a current resembling breath, and this displacement gives rise to the sensation of hearing.

Again, we must believe that smelling, like hearing, would produce no sensation, were there not particles conveyed from the object which are of the proper sort for exciting the organ of smelling, some of one sort, some of another, some exciting it confusedly and strangely, others quietly and agreeably.

Moreover, we must hold that the atoms in fact possess none of the qualities belonging to things which come under our observation, except shape, weight, and size, and the properties necessarily conjoined with shape. For every quality changes, but the atoms do not change, since, when the composite bodies are dissolved, there must needs be a permanent something, solid and indissoluble, left behind, which makes change possible: not changes into or from the non-existent. But often through differences of arrangement, and sometimes through additions and subtractions of the atoms. Hence these somethings capable of being diversely arranged must be indestructible, exempt from change, but possessed each of its own distinctive mass and configuration. This must remain.

For in the case of changes of configuration within our experience the figure is supposed to be inherent when other qualities are stripped of, but the qualities are not supposed, like the shape which is left behind, to inhere in the subject of change, but to vanish altogether from the body. Thus, then, what is left behind is sufficient to account for the differences in composite bodies, since something at least must necessarily be left remaining and be immune from annihilation.

Again, you should not suppose that the atoms have any and every size, lest you be contradicted by facts; but differences of size must be admitted; for this addition renders the facts of feeling and sensation easier of explanation. But to attribute any and every magnitude to the atoms does not help to explain the differences of quality in things; moreover, in that case atoms large enough to be seen ought to have reached us, which is never observed to occur; nor can we conceive how its occurrence should be possible, in other words that an atom should become visible.

Besides, you must not suppose that there are parts unlimited in number, be they ever so small, in any finite body. Hence not only must we reject as impossible subdivision ad infinitum into smaller and smaller parts, lest we make all things too weak and, in our conceptions of the aggregates, be driven to pulverize the things that exist, in other words the atoms, and annihilate them; but in dealing with finite things we must also reject as impossible the progression ad infinitum by less and less increments.

For when once we have said that an infinite number of particles, however small, are contained in anything, it is not possible to conceive how it could any longer be limited or finite in size. For clearly our infinite number of particles must have some size; and then, of whatever size they were, the aggregate they made would be infinite. And, in the next place, since what is finite has an extremity which is distinguishable, even if it is not by itself observable, it is not possible to avoid thinking of another such extremity next to this. Nor can we help thinking that in this way, by proceeding forward from one to the next in order, it is possible by such a progression to arrive in thought at infinity.

We must consider the minimum perceptible by sense as not corresponding to that which is capable of being traversed, that is to say is extended, nor again as utterly unlike it, but as having something in common with the things capable of being traversed, though it is without distinction of parts. But when from the illusion created by this common property we think we shall distinguish something in the minimum, one part on one side and another part on the other side, it must be another minimum equal to the first which catches our eye. In fact, we see these minima one after another, beginning with the first, and not as occupying the same space; nor do we see them touch one another's parts with their parts, but we see that by virtue of their own peculiar character (as being unit indivisibles) they afford a means of measuring magnitudes: there are more of them, if the magnitude measured is greater; fewer of them, if the magnitude measured is less.

We must recognize that this analogy also holds of the minimum in the atom; it is only in minuteness that it differs from that which is observed by sense, but it follows the same analogy. On the analogy of things within our experience we have declared that the atom has magnitude; and this, small as it is, we have merely reproduced on a larger scale. And further, the least and simplest things must be regarded as extremities of lengths, furnishing from themselves as units the means of measuring lengths, whether greater or less, the mental vision being employed, since direct observation is impossible. For the community which exists between them and the unchangeable parts (the minimal parts of area or surface) is sufficient to justify the conclusion so far as this goes. But it is not possible that these minima of the atom should group themselves together through the possession of motion.

Further, we must not assert "up" and "down" of that which is unlimited, as if there were a zenith or nadir. As to the space overhead, however, if it be possible to draw a line to infinity from the point where we stand, we know that never will this space—or, for that matter, the space below the supposed standpoint if produced to infinity—appear to us to be at the same time "up" and "down" with reference to the same point; for this is inconceivable. Hence it is possible to assume one direction of motion, which we conceive as extending upwards ad infinitum, and another downwards, even if it should happen ten thousand times that what moves from us to the spaces above our heads reaches the feet of those above us, or that which moves downwards from us the heads of those below us. None the less is it true that the whole of the motion in the respective cases is conceived as extending in opposite directions ad infinitum.

When they are traveling through the void and meet with no resistance, the atoms must move with equal speed. Neither will heavy atoms travel more quickly than small and light ones, so long as nothing meets them, nor will small atoms travel more quickly than large ones, provided they always find a passage suitable to their size. and provided also that they meet with no obstruction. Nor will their upward or their lateral motion, which is due to collisions, nor again their downward motion, due to weight, affect their velocity. As long as either motion obtains, it must continue, quick as the speed of thought, provided there is no obstruction, whether due to external collision or to the atoms' own weight counteracting the force of the blow.

Moreover, when we come to deal with composite bodies, one of them will travel faster than another, although their atoms have equal speed. This is because the atoms in the aggregates are traveling in one direction a during the shortest continuous time, albeit they move in different directions in times so short as to be appreciable only by the reason, but frequently collide until the continuity of their motion is appreciated by sense. For the assumption that beyond the range of direct observation even the minute times conceivable by reason will present continuity of motion is not true in the case before us. Our canon is that direct observation by sense and direct apprehension by the mind are alone invariably true.

Next, keeping in view our perceptions and feelings (for so shall we have the surest grounds for belief), we must recognize generally that the soul is a corporeal thing, composed of fine particles, dispersed all over the frame, most nearly resembling wind with an admixture of heat, in some respects like wind, in others like heat. But, again, there is the third part which exceeds the other two in the fineness of its particles and thereby keeps in closer touch with the rest of the frame. And this is shown by the mental faculties and feelings, by the ease with which the mind moves, and by thoughts, and by all those things the loss of which causes death. Further, we must keep in mind that soul has the greatest share in causing sensation. Still, it would not have had sensation, had it not been somehow confined within the rest of the frame. But the rest of the frame, though it provides this indispensable conditions for the soul, itself also has a share, derived from the soul, of the said quality; and yet does not possess all the qualities of soul. Hence on the departure of the soul it loses sentience. For it had not this power in itself; but something else, congenital with the body, supplied it to body: which other thing, through the potentiality actualized in it by means of motion, at once acquired for itself a quality of sentience, and, in virtue of the neighborhood and interconnection between them, imparted it (as I said) to the body also.

Hence, so long as the soul is in the body, it never loses sentience through the removal of some other part. The containing sheaths may be dislocated in whole or in part, and portions of the soul may thereby be lost; yet in spite of this the soul, if it manage to survive, will have sentience. But the rest of the frame, whether the whole of it survives or only a part, no longer has sensation, when once those atoms have departed, which, however few in number, are required to constitute the nature of soul. Moreover, when the whole frame is broken up, the soul is scattered and has no longer the same powers as before, nor the same notions; hence it does not possess sentience either.

For we cannot think of it as sentient, except it be in this composite whole and moving with these movements; nor can we so think of it when the sheaths which enclose and surround it are not the same as those in which the soul is now located and in which it performs these movements.

There is the further point to be considered, what the incorporeal can be, if, I mean, according to current usage the term is applied to what can be conceived as self-existent. But it is impossible to conceive anything that is incorporeal as self-existent except empty space. And empty space cannot itself either act or be acted upon, but simply allows body to move through it. Hence those who call soul incorporeal speak foolishly. For if it were so, it could neither act nor be acted upon. But, as it is, both these properties, you see, plainly belong to soul.

If, then, we bring all these arguments concerning soul to the criterion of our feelings and perceptions, and if we keep in mind the proposition stated at the outset, we shall see that the subject has been adequately comprehended in outline: which will enable us to determine the details with accuracy and confidence.

Moreover, shapes and colors, magnitudes and weights, and in short all those qualities which are predicated of body, in so far as they are perpetual properties either of all bodies or of visible bodies, are knowable by sensation of these very properties: these, I say, must not be supposed to exist independently by themselves (for that is inconceivable), nor yet to be non-existent, nor to be some other and incorporeal entities cleaving to body, nor again to be parts of body. We must consider the whole body in a general way to derive its permanent nature from all of them, though it is not, as it were, formed by grouping them together in the same way as when from the particles themselves a larger aggregate is made up, whether these particles be primary or any magnitudes whatsoever less than the particular whole. All these qualities, I repeat, merely give the body its own permanent nature. They all have their own characteristic modes of being perceived and distinguished, but always along with the whole body in which they inhere and never in separation from it; and it is in virtue of this complete conception of the body as a whole that it is so designated.

Again, qualities often attach to bodies without being permanent concomitants. They are not to be classed among invisible entities nor are they incorporeal. Hence, using the term "accidents" in the commonest sense, we say plainly that "accidents" have not the nature of the whole thing to which they belong, and to which, conceiving it as a whole, we give the name of body, nor that of the permanent properties without which body cannot be thought of. And in virtue of certain peculiar modes of apprehension into which the complete body always enters, each of them can be called an accident. But only as often as they are seen actually to belong to it, since such accidents are not perpetual concomitants. There is no need to banish from reality this clear evidence that the accident has not the nature of that whole—by us called body—to which it belongs, nor of the permanent properties which accompany the whole. Nor, on the other hand, must we suppose the accident to have independent existence (for this is just as inconceivable in the case of accidents as in that of the permanent properties); but, as is manifest, they should all be regarded as accidents, not as permanent concomitants, of bodies, nor yet as having the rank of independent existence. Rather they are seen to be exactly as and what sensation itself makes them individually claim to be.

There is another thing which we must consider carefully. We must not investigate time as we do the other accidents which we investigate in a subject, namely, by referring them to the preconceptions envisaged in our minds; but we must take into account the plain fact itself, in virtue of which we speak of time as long or short, linking to it in intimate connection this attribute of duration. We need not adopt any fresh terms as preferable, but should employ the usual expressions about it. Nor need we predicate anything else of time, as if this something else contained the same essence as is contained in the proper meaning of the word "time" (for this also is done by some). We must chiefly reflect upon that to which we attach this peculiar character of time, and by which we measure it. No further proof is required: we have only to reflect that we attach the attribute of time to days and nights and their parts, and likewise to feelings of pleasure and pain and to neutral states, to states of movement and states of rest, conceiving a peculiar accident of these to be this very characteristic which we express by the word "time."

After the foregoing we have next to consider that the worlds and every finite aggregate which bears a strong resemblance to things we commonly see have arisen out of the infinite. For all these, whether small or great, have been separated off from special conglomerations of atoms; and all things are again dissolved, some faster, some slower, some through the action of one set of causes, others through the action of another.

And further, we must not suppose that the worlds have necessarily one and the same shape. For nobody can prove that in one sort of world there might not be contained, whereas in another sort of world there could not possibly be, the seeds out of which animals and plants arise and all the rest of the things we see.

Again, we must suppose that nature too has been taught and forced to learn many various lessons by the facts themselves, that reason subsequently develops what it has thus received and makes fresh discoveries, among some tribes more quickly, among others more slowly, the progress thus made being at certain times and seasons greater, at others less.

Hence even the names of things were not originally due to convention, but in the several tribes under the impulse of special feelings and special presentations of sense primitive man uttered special cries. The air thus emitted was molded by their individual feelings or sense-presentations, and differently according to the difference of the regions which the tribes inhabited. Subsequently whole tribes adopted their own special names, in order that their communications might be less ambiguous to each other and more briefly expressed. And as for things not visible, so far as those who were conscious of them tried to introduce any such notion, they put in circulation certain names for them, either sounds which they were instinctively compelled to utter or which they selected by reason on analogy according to the most general cause there can be for expressing oneself in such a way.

Nay more: we are bound to believe that in the sky revolutions, solstices, eclipses, risings and settings, and the like, take place without the ministration or command, either now or in the future, of any being who it the same time enjoys perfect bliss along with immortality. For troubles and anxieties and feelings of anger and partiality do not accord with bliss, but always imply weakness and fear and dependence upon one's neighbors. Nor, again, must we hold that things which are no more than globular masses of fire, being at the same time endowed with bliss, assume these motions at will. Nay, in every term we use we must hold fast to all the majesty which attaches to such notions as bliss and immortality, lest the terms should generate opinions inconsistent with this majesty. Otherwise such inconsistency will of itself suffice to produce the worst disturbance in our minds. Hence, where we find phenomena invariably recurring, the invariability of the recurrence must be ascribed to the original interception and conglomeration of atoms whereby the world was formed.

Further, we must hold that to arrive at accurate knowledge of the cause of things of most moment is the business of natural science, and that happiness depends on this (viz. on the knowledge of celestial and atmospheric phenomena), and upon knowing what the heavenly bodies really are, and any kindred facts contributing to exact knowledge in this respect.

Further, we must recognize on such points as this no plurality of causes or contingency, but must hold that nothing suggestive of conflict or disquiet is compatible with an immortal and blessed nature. And the mind can grasp the absolute truth of this.

But when we come to subjects for special inquiry, there is nothing in the knowledge of risings and settings and solstices and eclipses and all kindred subjects that contributes to our happiness; but those who are well-informed about such matters and yet are ignorant—what the heavenly bodies really are, and what are the most important causes of phenomena, feel quite as much fear as those who have no such special information—nay, perhaps even greater fear, when the curiosity excited by this additional knowledge cannot find a solution or understand the subordination of these phenomena to the highest causes.

Hence, if we discover more than one cause that may account for solstices, settings and risings, eclipses and the like, as we did also in particular matters of detail, we must not suppose that our treatment of these matters fails of accuracy, so far as it is needful to ensure our tranquility and happiness. When, therefore, we investigate the causes of celestial and atmospheric phenomena, as of all that is unknown, we must take into account the variety of ways in which analogous occurrences happen within our experience; while as for those who do not recognize the difference between what is or comes about from a single cause and that which may be the effect of any one of several causes, overlooking the fact that the objects are only seen at a distance, and are moreover ignorant of the conditions that render, or do not render, peace of mind impossible—all such persons we must treat with contempt. If then we think that an event could happen in one or other particular way out of several, we shall be as tranquil when we recognize that it actually comes about in more ways than one as if we knew that it happens in this particular way.

There is yet one more point to seize, namely, that the greatest ,anxiety of the human mind arises through the belief that the heavenly bodies are blessed and indestructible, and that at the same time they have volition and actions and causality inconsistent with this belief; and through expecting or apprehending some everlasting evil, either because of the myths, or because we are in dread of the mere insensibility of death, as if it had to do with us; and through being reduced to this state not by conviction but by a certain irrational perversity, so that, if men do not set bounds to their terror, they endure as much or even more intense anxiety than the man whose views on these matters are quite vague. But mental tranquility means being released from all these troubles and cherishing a continual remembrance of the highest and most important truths.

Hence we must attend to present feelings and sense perceptions, whether those of mankind in general or those peculiar to the individual, and also attend to all the clear evidence available, as given by each of the standards of truth. For by studying them we shall rightly trace to its cause and banish the source of disturbance and dread, accounting for celestial phenomena and for all other things which from time to time befall us and cause the utmost alarm to the rest of mankind.

Here then, Herodotus, you have the chief doctrines of Physics in the form of a summary. So that, if this statement be accurately retained and take effect, a man will, I make no doubt, be incomparably better equipped than his fellows, even if he should never go into all the exact details. For he will clear up for himself many of the points which I have worked out in detail in my complete exposition; and the summary itself, if borne in mind, will be of constant service to him.

It is of such a sort that those who are already tolerably, or even perfectly, well acquainted with the details can, by analysis of what they know into such elementary perceptions as these, best prosecute their researches in physical science as a whole; while those, on the other hand, who are not altogether entitled to rank as mature students can in silent fashion and as quick as thought run over the doctrines most important for their peace of mind.

ANNEX 5

THE BIOGRAPHY OF EPICURUS

"Epicurus, son of Neocles and Chaerestrate, was an Athenian of the Gargets ward and the Philaidae clan, as Metrodorus says in his book On Noble Birth. He is said by Heraclides (in his Epitome of Sotion) as well as by others, to have been brought up at Samos after the Athenians had sent colonists there, and to have come to Athens at the age of eighteen, at the time when Xenocrates was head of the Academy and Aristotle was in Chalcis. After the death of Alexander of Macedon and the expulsion of the Athenian colonists from Samos by Perdiccas, Epicurus left Athens to join his father in Colophon; for some time he stayed there and gathered students around him, then returned to Athens again during the archonship of Anaxicrates." (Diogenes Laertius).

Epicurus' parents transmitted to him the democratic spirit, while his experience of the disasters that Athens suffered from the aristocracy and the militaristic regimes influenced him to see life from the point of view of the common man, in contrast with the famous aristocrat sages, Plato and Aristotle. In Samos he was taught by Nausiphanes, and the Platonic Pamphilus. As the island was under the influence of the Ionian naturalistic culture, Epicurus soon moved away from the Platonic beliefs and turned to the materialistic theories of Democritus. At the age of eighteen he was drafted into the Athenian army, where he met his intimate friend, the dramatic poet Menander.

Little is known of his life during the following fifteen years. What is known, though, is that he created his own philosophical circle in Mytilene and then in Lampsacus. He returned to Athens in around 307 BC at the age of thirty four to buy a piece of land between Athens and Piraeus, close to the present Agronomic School. There he housed his philosophical school, which he named "The Garden." Epicurus taught there for thirty-five years, following a simple life, surrounded by men, women, courtesans and slaves, who participated equally in the Epicurean Garden. He died when he was seventy-one years old, in 270 BC.

During the Hellenistic period the dominant philosophical schools were the Epicurean and the Stoic, followed by the Platonic, the Aristotelian, the Skeptics and the Cynics. The principles of the Epicurean Philosophy spread throughout the Greek and the Roman world from the Epicurean school of philosophy in Athens. Epicurus was among the most prolific philosophers in history. He authored works, developed in 300 rolls, the fate of which has been ignored ever since the proclamation of Christianity as the official religion of the Byzantine Empire. Through Diogenes Laertius, a biographer of philosophers of the 3rd century AD, three of his letters survived (to Herodotus, On Nature, to Pythocles, On Celestial Bodies and to Menoeceus, On Ethics), as well as his Will and the Principal Doctrines, which is a summary of his philosophy.

Ponzio Bratziolini also discovered the poem De Rerum Natura (On the Nature of Things) of the Roman Epicurean philosopher-poet Lucretius (94-55 BC), in a German monastery, in 1414 AD. The poem is developed over six books and contains the Epicurean views on Nature. In 1884, two French archaeologists discovered the great inscription of the Epicurean Diogenes Oenoanda in Ionia, Asia Minor, which is considered a grand philosophical monument of humanity. A collection of Epicurean doctrines named Vatican Sayings was found at the

Vatican in 1888. Opinions on the Epicurean Philosophy were identified in the works of many writers, Athenaeus, Cicero, Seneca, Sextus Empiricus, Plutarch, and so on. Also, new texts are still coming to light from the charred papyri of an ancient villa that was destroyed by the eruption of Vesuvius, close to the city of Herculaneum in Italy.

Intellectuals in the period of the Enlightenment embraced the Epicurean principles and spread them around the world. An eminent figure of world history, Thomas Jefferson (1743-1826), the third President of the USA (1801-1809) and leading author of the Declaration of Independence, wrote in his letter to William Short: "As you say of yourself, I too am an Epicurean... Their [the Stoics] great crime was in their calumnies of Epicurus and misrepresentations of his doctrines..."

Today, both in Greece and globally, the Epicurean Philosophy is followed and spread by the modern Epicureans according to Epicurus' will: "Farewell my friends, the truths I taught hold fast." The Epicurean Philosophy laid the foundations for individual and materialist metaphysical views of the universe. It was a source of inspiration for Marx, as we can conclude from the topic of his doctoral thesis, Difference between the Democritean and Epicurean Philosophy of Nature. Although initially Marx applauded the Epicurean views, he later embraced the Stoic ideas of Hegel, and suggested the pursuance of duty in the context of destiny as the end of life, according to the stoic philosophy, instead of the pursuit of pleasure.

The spread of the Epicurean teaching in antiquity owes to its practical spirit, according to which philosophy is not an end in itself, but a means and an aid in achieving the objective of human life, which is happiness. Therefore Epicurus did not give any importance to extensive theoretical, grammatical, historical and mathematical research if it did not contribute to living happily. On the other hand, he attributed the malaise of the people to ignorance and superstition, and proposed the knowledge and application of the laws that govern the nature of the cosmos and human beings as a cure.

Afterword

Being absorbed for several months in researching the uncomfortable subject of death has turned out to be a worthwhile adventure. Taming the fear of death proved to be both liberating and revitalizing. I hope that you too will be relieved by assimilating the therapeutic arguments and practices presented in the lines of this monograph.

Common wisdom advocates that gazing into death is dreadful and therefore should be renounced. It moreover advises taking advantage of a wide spectrum of defensive mechanisms ranging from societal and cultural to religious and personal, such as raising children, being creative, pursuing wealth, fame, and power. To our disappointment, these vehicles may be beneficial in the short term, but over the long run they manifest hurting secondary effects that undermine the quality of our life and procure painful mental illnesses.

Contrary to the compelling presence of the denial of death in everyday life, the Epicurean philosophy and contemporary psychology alike encourage a full unwavering look at the subject. They deliver convincing evidence that reveals the so-called terror of death to be pointless as it is unmoved by the intellect and indifferent to our anxiety and trepidation, since once dead our entire being dissolves into its constituent atoms driving both consciousness and soul into nothingness. Therefore, for no reason at all should we worry about something that when it happens is nothingness. Besides, the idea that death will deprive us of the good things in life is preposterous since we will never sense any kind of loss. To our surprise then, the appalling fear of death is, after all, the most absurd fear ever experienced by man. Its widespread presence stems from the false societal and cultural beliefs supporting that either we will feel the loss of our life or suffer the torments of Hell. Quite the reverse, the truth is that the evil is not death, but pain. It consequently deserves to readjust our beliefs by establishing pleasure-pain as the guide to our life rather than the fear of death.

Through many months of intense research, I gradually convinced myself that facing the fear of death is not a hard task to take on. Reversely, it is a straightforward reaction to challenge and degrade it to the level of a fantastical-unrealistic fear; the terror of death can be scaled down to everyday manageable anxiety through the mediation of philosophical arguments and practices. Glaring into the face of death, with philosophical counseling, puts an end to the terror and generates a more touching, more valuable, and more joyful life. We should meditate our terminal finale with the helping hand of the teachings of Epicurus and contemporary scientific findings: by seizing our human nature—our mortality, our transience in the light—we will come to treasure the grandeur of each moment and the pleasure of sheer existence.

Tension and uneasiness will always go together with our encounter with death. I am conscious of it now as I put in writing these phrases; it is the cost we bear for self-awareness. But I guarantee you, it is worthwhile embarking on this lifesaving enterprise.